AVICENNA'S POEM ON MEDICINE

AVICENNA'S POEM
ON
MEDICINE

By

HAVEN C. KRUEGER, A.M., M.D.
Wichita, Kansas

With a Foreword by

Ralph H. Major, M.D.
Library of the History of Medicine
University of Kansas Medical School
Kansas City, Kansas

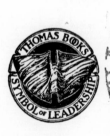

C H A R L E S   C   T H O M A S · P U B L I S H E R
Springfield · Illinois · U.S.A.

Published and Distributed Throughout the World by
CHARLES C THOMAS · PUBLISHER
BANNERSTONE HOUSE
301-327 East Lawrence Avenue, Springfield, Illinois, U.S.A.

© *1963, by* CHARLES C THOMAS · PUBLISHER
Library of Congress Catalog Card Number: 62-17607

With THOMAS BOOKS careful attention is given to all details of manufacturing and design. It is the Publisher's desire to present books that are satisfactory as to their physical qualities and artistic possibilities and appropriate for their particular use. THOMAS BOOKS will be true to those laws of quality that assure a good name and good will.

Printed in the United States of America

For her many hours of generous and gracious aid during the compilation of this writing, devoted appreciation and gratitude are expressed to my wife, Ruby N. Krueger, to whom this *opus parvus* is affectionately dedicated.

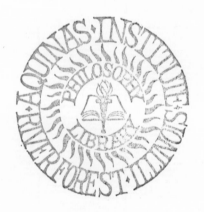

Foreword

A VICENNA, described by Osler as "the author of the most famous medical text-book ever written," was also one of the greatest poets Islam has produced. He summarized his medical knowledge in a series of poems—cantica. While the Canon and the Cantica were translated into Latin by Gerard of Cremona in the Twelfth Century, English translations of these two classics have waited until the twentieth century to appear.

In 1930, O. Cameron Gruner made an English translation of the first fen of the Canon, with notes, directly from the Arabic. An announcement has been made that an English translation of the whole Canon by M. H. Shah is to appear in 1962. This translation by Dr. Krueger appears to be the first English translation of the Cantica. He based it primarily on a French version with frequent references to German and Latin sources. We are sure this work will be welcomed by all students and physicians interested in the history of medicine.

RALPH H. MAJOR, M.D.

Preface

*N*OT ONLY is it impossible to render adequately an exact transcription of thoughts composed a millenium ago but also it is impossible to convey percisely contextual meaning, Oriental imagery and poetic beauty. Such is what this author has encountered in his endeavor to supply the monolingual American physician with an intelligible interpretation of the *'Arjuzat fi't-tibb (Poem on Medicine)* of Avicenna. Although modern Arabic grammar differs only slightly from that of medieval Oriental writers, Arabic semantics during the past thousand years have not remained static.

While it was this author's primary objective merely to offer a translation of the recently published French version (26), the occasional doubt which has arisen from time to time concerning the exactitude of the rendition into French of the *Poème sur la médecine* has caused this author to rely somewhat heavily on the German *Lehrgedicht über die Heilkunde* (36) and on the Latin *Canticum avicennae* (26). It has even been necessary to undertake the study of elementary Arabic so that some of the original words could be expressed more aptly in the English version presented in this paper.

H. C. K.

Acknowledgments

*T*HE AUTHOR is indebted to Miss Phoebe Peck and Doctor R. H. Major for the encouragement in undertaking this task; to Miss Peck and Miss Emma Lue Kopp for their valuable assistance in locating obscure source materials necessary for the thoroughness of this investigation.

Contents

AVICENNA'S POEM ON MEDICINE

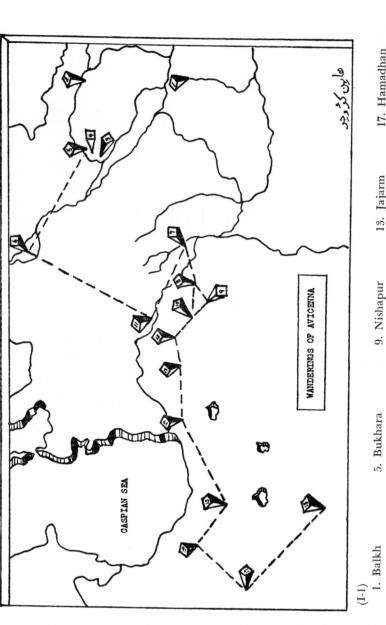

(1-1)

1. Balkh
2. Samarkand
3. Afshena
4. Kharmaithan

5. Bukhara
6. Gurganj
7. Baward
8. Tus

9. Nishapur
10. Shaqqan
11. Fasa
12. Samanqan

13. Jajarm
14. Jurjan
15. Raiy
16. Qazwin

17. Hamadhan
18. Isfahan

WANDERINGS OF AVICENNA

CASPIAN SEA

1

Avicenna, His Life and Works

*T*HE ELDER of two sons born in August 980 (Ṣafar 370
A. H.) (1-2) * to 'Abd-Allāh, the local govenor of Kharmaithan of Isma'ili origin and his wife, Sittare, from
Afshena, of Persian descent, was Abū 'Alī al-Ḥusain ibn
'Abd-Allāh ibn Ḥasan ibn 'Ali ibn Sīnā (I-3) who through
the Europeanized Hebrew transliteration of his name has
become known to us as Avicenna.

After five years of age, Avicenna's formative years were
spent in Bukhārā, his father's permanent home, with his
family in a liberal religious atmosphere. By the age of ten
he had memorized the *Qur'an* as well as a few other philosophical writings. Because of his remarkable talent, his
father sent him to a local merchant to learn Indian arith-
metic at which same time Avicenna was also studying
Muslim jurisprudence and acquiring methods of religious
argumentation from an old ascetic of Bukhārā. With the
help of al-Natheli whom Avicenna's father employed, the
young pupil was guided through elementary logic, Por-
phyry's *Isagoge,* Euclid, and Ptolemy's *Almagest.* Avicenna
continued his studies in natural sciences and metaphysics,
mostly of Plato and Aristotle, in the original with aid from
commentaries of Hellenistic authors translated into Arabic
after his teacher left.

About the age of sixteen Avicenna acquired a desire to
pursue medicine and he read every available book on the
subject, finding this science not difficult.

---

*All simple numbers in parenthesis, i.e. (26), refer directly to biblio-
graphical entries whereas compound numbers, i.e. (I-1), refer to the notes
of the various sections.

His philosophical problems were solved through prayers and endless hard work and strengthened by wine, he never rested during the next two years. Avicenna endeavored to understand Aristotle's *Metaphysica* through forty laborious readings, but only with the aid of al-Farabi's commentary was the young Persian able to assimilate the material.

At this time, Nūh ibn Mansūr, the ruling prince, became ill and his physicians, unable to cure the monarch, suggested that Avicenna be summoned. Soon Avicenna had cured the prince who repaid his gratitude by allowing the young scholar access to the library of the Sāmānid rulers. Later, when this library burned, Avicenna's enemies were eager to point an accusing finger at their erudite superior.

At twenty-one years of age, while still in Bukhārā, the philosopher-physician tried his hand at writing, answering requests of certain friends. He was successful in completing the *Majmū'* (Compendium), a comprehensive book on the science and art of versification, the twenty volume *al-Ḥāsil wa al-Maḥṣūl* (the Import and the Substance), dealing with jurisprudence, and a work on ethics *al-Birr wa al-Ithm* (Good Work and Evil).

A year later when his father died, Avicenna accepted a post (type unknown) with Sulṭān Maḥmūd of Gurganj as a source of income. The young Persian was royally welcomed, but soon obscure circumstances caused him to leave this city.

In the next few years, wanderings led Avicenna to Fasā, Bāward, Ṭūs, Shaqqān, Samanqān, Jājarm and Jurjān. It was in 1013 in Jurjān that Jūzjānī became Avicenna's closest companion, biographer and secretary. In this town, Avicenna began composing *al-Qānūn* (the Canon) (I-4), an admirable tome which induced his contemporaries to grant him the title of *al-Sheikh al-Ra'is* (the Chief, the

Teacher) and a century later provoked Latin scholiasts to call him *Medicorum Principes* (the Prince of Physicians) (I-5).

For indefinite reasons, Avicenna and Jūzjānī chose to journey to Raiy in which the young but mature philosopher was welcomed by Princess al-Saiyyida and her son, Majd al-Dowlah. During the next three years, the Prince of Physicians composed the *Kitāb al-Ma'ād* (Book of the Return) and created such dissensions between the two monarchs that he was obliged to leave Raiy.

The philosopher, his brother and his faithful companion traveled to Qazwīn and from there, went to Hamadhān. It was in 1024 in Hamadhān that Avicenna assumed an active rôle in politics. Through the influence of a lady (I-6), the maturing Persian became acquainted with the ruler, Shams al-Dowlah and cured him from an attack of colic. He soon won the favor of the Amir, accompanied the latter during a military expedition as a personal physician, and on their return to Hamadhān was appointed vizier. His first attempt as state administrator failed because of the army's dislike of the philosopher-physician. Avicenna was forced into hiding, but was soon called to cure Shams al-Dowlah of colic; the Amir then reappointed the physician as vizier.

Although his daylight hours were devoted to political affairs, Avicenna's nights were occupied with writing, group discussions and the pleasures of wine, women and music. At this time, the Prince of Physicians continued work on *al-Qānūn* and began his *Kitāb al-Shifā* (Book of Healing), the longest of his extant works, and completed *al-Adwiyat al-Qalbiyya* (the Remedies of the Heart).

Following the death of the Amir, Avicenna secretly offered his services to 'Alā al-Dowlah, ruler of Iṣfahān. Shams al-Dowlah learned of this correspondence and through Avicenna's enemies, imprisoned the philosopher. Avicenna was not idle in captivity before his release by the conquering army of 'Alā al-Dowlah. During those four months, he continued the *Kitāb al-Shifā* and wrote the *Kitāb al-Hidāya* (Book of Guidance), *Risālat Haiyibn Yaqzān* (Treatise on Living, the Son of the Vigilant), and *Kitāb al-Qulanj* (Book of Colic).

Under the patronage of 'Alā al-Dowlah in Iṣfahān, Avicenna conducted scientific and philosophical meetings, composed *Dānish-Nāmeh ye' Alā'i* ('Alā'i Book of Knowledge), dedicated to his patron, finished *Kitāb al Shifā*, compiled an abridgement of the latter work, *Kitāb al-Najāt* (Book of Deliverance), studied Arabic grammar and literature, delved into linguistics, summarizing his observations in *Lisān al'Arab* (Language of the Arabs), and wrote *Kitāb al-Inṣaf* (Book of Equitable Judgment).

The fall of Raiy to the army of the Sulṭan Maḥmūd endangered the position of 'Alā al-Dowlah in Iṣfahān. This ruler fled in the company of Avicenna and at this time, the Prince of Physicians developed an inopportune case of colic followed by epilepsy. Avicenna tried to cure himself with multiple abdominal injections which only served to provoke intestinal ulceration. The philosopher-physician was carried to Iṣfahān where he improved somewhat, but he continued to indulge in licentious living, pleasures which ultimately undermined his intrinsically strong constitution.

Once, again, the Prince of Physicians accompanied 'Alā al-Dowlah during the latter's march on Hamadhān. Before reaching that city, Avicenna suffered a severe relapse of the colic. He remained in a state of ill-health and shortly after he arrived at Hamadhān, the Prince of Physicians died on the last Friday night of the month of

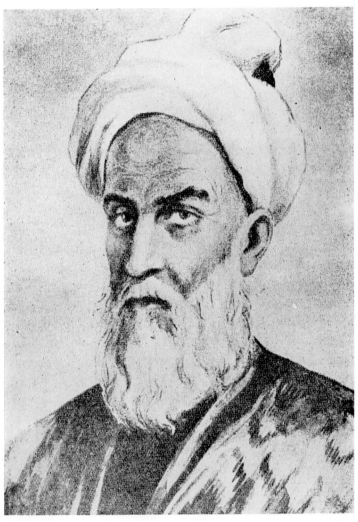

Avicenna at the end of his life. (According to an authorized painting
by the artist W. Wysockiego.) (15)

Ramadhān 428 A. H. (1037 A. D.) in his 58th year of life (I-7).

It is certain that Avicenna's fame rests as much upon his medical writings as upon his metaphysical compositions which outnumbered his scientific endeavors (8, 31, 39). He is credited with about one hundred works in Arabic and Persian of which the most important ones are still extant (1). It is interesting to note that the philosopher-physician's compositions contain a fascinating and varied language although he was never considered a real literary individual (1, 4).

Al-Qānūn is by far his major contribution to medicine, containing about a million words, which served as a medical bible for a longer period of time than any other work (1, 31, 37). Although a discussion of this encyclopedia is beyond the scope of this book, this large work demonstrated the Chief Master's enthusiasm for the use of the *mot juste,* one word with only one meaning, and for succinct classification, both of which serve to give some insight into his personality (1, 44).

Avicenna is also known in the medical world for his infinitesimally smaller work *al-'Arjuzat fi't-tibb* (the Poem on Medicine) which has enjoyed a Western as well as Eastern position equal to that of *al-Qānūn* (13, 17, 26, 27, 29, 47).

Bridging the gap between the Eastern and Western civilizations, Avicenna stands among the prominent men of history; he has even been counted by Dante in *Inferno* among the greatest minds of the non-Christian world (I-8).

Although his medical experience was transcendentally greater than that of Galen, it is evident that Avicenna had Hellenistic, Byzantine, Persian and Arabic sources span-

ning eight and one-half centuries from which to draw
(44). Nevertheless, some authorities state that the Prince
of Physicians demonstrated a mind like Goethe's, possessed
a genius similar to that of Leonardo da Vinci (32, 43), and
revealed a dynamic personality filled with an insatiable
desire to acquire knowledge as well as with serenity and
sensitivity (50). It is clear that no Muslim or Oriental
scholar has attained as high a position and has held as
strong and enduring an influence as Avicenna has in the
history of the World (44).

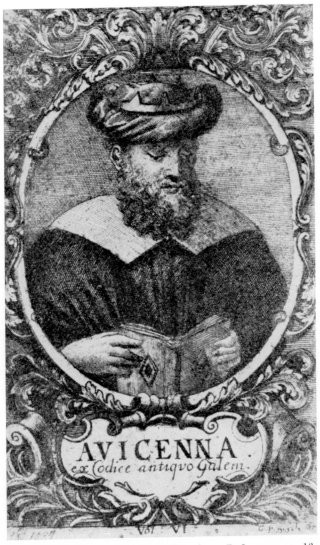

An old woodcut of Avicenna taken from Reference no. 13.

2

History of The Poem on Medicine

*B*ESIDE *al-Qānūn*, Avicenna's work most frequently found throughout Europe is *al-' Arjuzat fi'ṭ-ṭibb* (the Poem on Medicine) (29). This undated compendium is an abridgement of the ideas presented within *al-Qānūn* and is considered by some authorities to be the most widely read (47) and of almost equal value with the *opus magnus* (13, 16, 29) although other authors only mention the *Poem* in passing (9, 17, 28). One Arabist enthusiastically and dogmatically states that there is hardly a medical work "the vogue of which may be compared to that enjoyed by the great poem of Avicenna" (40). One of the few comments from this continent adds that Avicenna's *opus parvus* merits more than fleeting attention of the students of medieval medicine (47). Avenzoar, who held little regard for *al-Qānūn,* proclaimed that the principles of science which the *Poem* contains make this work more valuable than a whole library of books (29).

Al-'Arjuzat fi'ṭ-ṭibb was known in Western cultures during the middle ages in its translations (27). The first extant indication of this work's having been translated into a European language was that done by Gerardo of Cremona who lived between 1114 and 1187, placing this rendition sometime in the middle of the twelfth century (10). A century later, Armengaud de Blaise of Montpellier included a Latin translation of the *Poem* along with the works of Averroes; although the date of this work was probably 1281 (27), inclusive dates from one year before that up to eight years after that have been suggested (3, 22).

9

Between 1520 and 1522, a publication appeared in Venice with Blaise's *Poem,* Averroes' comments and a complete translation of *al-Qānūn* to which were added the comments of Gentile, Jacques Desparts, Johannes Mattheus Gradi, and Thadea of Florence. The *Poem* was published without the comments in Lyon in 1522, the author of which was Pierre Antoine Rusticus dofe Plaisance. In this edition, the author omitted the comments but corrected the style and errors and included an index of useful Arabic terms (27).

Yet another series of translations of the *Poem* was begun by Andrea Alpagus of Bellune who added his efforts with the publication of 1527. This work and the ones which followed apparently did not include Averroes' comments. In 1562, Benedictus Rinius Venetus introduced marginal notes to clarify many points of poorly indicated Avicennisms while in 1608 Joanne Costus and Joanne Paulo Mongius contributed an index and vocabulary (27).

The only translation of this *Poem* into verse was completed in the sixteenth century by Jean Faucher, but this work was not printed until 1630 in the Nîmes' edition of Guillaume Faucher. Both this publication and that of Antonius Deusingius demonstrate considerable contextual deviation from the translation of Alpagus (27).

In 1649 appeared the last prose edition in Latin written by Antonius Deusingius and published in Groningue. It is obvious that this Arabist had access to all the previous translations so that his should reflect all the good qualities of previous attempts. Investigators claim that Deusingius was the only one who included an approximation of the Arabic text of the *Poem's* preface in verse. It is true that all of the works prior to 1649 are valuable, but Deusingius' is of incomparable value because it follows most closely the Arabic text, rarely deviating from the exact sense of the words and then only in a justifiable manner (27).

In general, it is easily understood how numerous errors might have crept into all of the translations when one considers that the copyists of the Arabic texts were probably not meticulous with their transcriptions of already indistinctly written material. In addition, the translators themselves were guilty of too literal a rendition of terms or transcribed them phonetically and even went through the Arabic to original Hellenistic sources (27).

Al'-Arjuzat fi't-tibb falls into the category of the literary *genre* known as didactic poetry which ultimately expires in the hands of scholars, being minutely dissected and discussed word by word. Thus, it happened that there were five individuals known to have executed such a dissection of the *Poem*. It is agreed that Ibn Rushd, better known in Western culture as Averroes, was the first to study Avicenna's small work thoroughly in the middle twelfth century. Following him were a student of the Hispanized Muslim's Ibn Tumulūs, Ibn Muḥammad, *ca.* 1386 A. D., Ibn al-Muhannā, early fifteenth century, and in the Orient, al-Ṣakālli, also early fifteenth century (40).

As for the actual literary mechanics on which Avicenna built his *'Arjuzat,* little has been written. It would probably be necessary to resort to a study of Averroes' comments to obtain a true appreciation of the poetry as seen through medieval eyes. Nevertheless, it is generally recognized that the poem was written with simplicity in mind to which *rajaz* meter leads itself well (II-1).

Only within the last twenty-five years may it be stated that Avicenna's *'Arjuzat* has followed the majority of Arabic translations in that they have been published mainly in French and German (23). It is through the publica-

tions of Jahier and Noureddine, Opitz and Deusingius
(26, 36) that the following English interpretation of the
Poem on Medicine has been made possible.

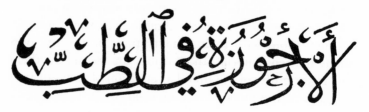

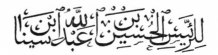

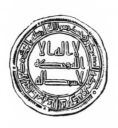

اعتنى بنشر نصها العربي ونص ترجمتها
اللاتينية وقام بنقلها الى اللغة الفرنسية
الدكتو جان جاهي والشيخ عبد القادر نور الدين
الاستاذان بجامعة الجزائر
باريس
١٣٧٥ — ١٩٥٦

Title page of the *Poem* in Arabic found in Reference no. 26.

3

The Poem on Medicine

Preface in Prose

*T*HE SHEIKH, the Prince of Physicians, 'Abū 'Alī al-Ḥusain Ibn 'Abd Allāh Ibn Sīnā stated:

It was customary for philosophers and men of knowledge of ancient times to serve kings, amirs, caliphs, viziers, judges and jurists by drawing up for them writings in prose and poetry, volumes consecrated to the arts and sciences and especially medical poems.

As for physicians, they often write poems in *rajaz* and make collections which permit us to distinguish the eloquent man from the one who is not, the skillful from the incompetent. Thus, it is that kings became acquainted with the precepts of medicine and philosophical methods.

I have seen that in certain countries medical art did not promote discussion meetings, nor polemics, as much in hospitals as in schools; I have seen people, unprovided with a scientific foundation, without any idea of its laws and deprived of any ethical formation, busy themselves with medicine without having studied it. Thus, men without thorough knowledge have pushed themselves forward and have considered themselves teachers. Now, I cast myself upon the footsteps of the ancients and the philosophers and I have served his Excellency, our Majesty the Vizier, the Jurist, the Judge, the Illustrious, whose position is exalted (may Allah prolong his life, allow his power and his glory to continue and overthrow his jealous subjects and his enemies) ; I have served him with this *'Arjuzat,* a poem which deals with every part of medicine.

13

I have divided this *'Arjuzat* in a remarkable manner; I have dressed it with a complete raiment and adorned it with a gown of beauty.

It is drawn up in a very simple style, in convenient versification, so that it may be easy, less difficult to understand.

When Our Majesty looks at it with all his acuteness of mind and it takes a place among his books in a small form, he will make use of it in order to acquire this magnificent science. Then, he will know how to discern the true practitioner from the despicable mob, the apprentice from the perfect savant, and the erudite from the blockhead.

I beseech Allah to help me in one of those works which bring us nearer to Him and lift their author to His eyes.

It is from Him that I beg His help and in Him that I place my confidence.

Preface in Verse

Praise be to Allah, the Teacher, the Unique, Majesty of the Heavens, the Exalted, the Glorious. Glory be to Him, the Eternal Being who drew forth creatures from Nothingness. He floods our minds with light to the point of having revealed to them that which was hidden. In His goodness, He created man and gave him judgment and speech as privileges. He allowed him access to knowledge through the perceptions of his senses and, through reasoning, opened to him the invisible world. The mind of man is bound to a living soul of which the existence is proved beyond all doubt. Allah distributed judgment and senses among all men at the same time as life. But each one has his own character and in that His Marvellous Wisdom shines forth. Thus, whoever has banished Ugliness from his soul has been able to acquire Virtue. The arts and speech distinguish man from animal. The best of men do good by accompanying it with courteous words, preoccupying themselves with the body, granting to it its rightful mirth. Poets are the princes of the Word; physicians rule over the Body. The eloquence of the former rejoices the soul; the devotion of the latter cures illnesses. In this poem is included all Theoretical and Practical Medicine. And here I am, putting into verse all I know of this science.

On the definition of the word "Medicine"

Medicine is the preservation of health and the cure of disease which arises from conscious causes which exist within the body.

Subdivision of Medicine

A first division will be: Theory and Practice. Theory within itself is divided into three sections. There are seven natural components and six vital factors. Indeed, they are found in books. They are the diseases, the symptoms and the causes. Practice is divided into two actions: one performed with the hands, the other with medicine and dietary regimens.

On the natural components and first about the Elements

The elements are the constitutive factors of bodies. The opinion of Hippocrates on the subject of the elements is accurate; there are four of them: water, fire, earth, air. The proof of the accuracy of this notion is that after death, the body returns to them through necessity. Moreover, if it were composed of only a single element, one would not know how to observe any living being touched by illness.

Second natural component—Temperaments

After that, perfect knowledge of the temperaments aids in the treatment of illness. The temperament has four

aspects which the physician will separate or join together.
It may be warm, cold, dry or moist, expressions perceptible
by touch. These qualities are found in the elements
(III-1), in the seasons, in the kingdoms (III-2), and in
places. The raw material is the primordial constitutive
source of bodies. Warmth is in fire and air, cold in earth
and water, dryness between fire and earth, moisture between water and air. These qualities are also found in the
elements which are of different natures and which make
up bodies by their arrangements. These qualities are different in that there will be only one and they group themselves without opposing each other (III-3). We have an
idea of the temperament of someone because of this ar-
rangement of elements and thus, we give him the classification of that which predominates. The temperament is
said to be balanced when it includes the four qualities.
They exist in man according to certain proportions which
serve as a pattern and model. Every man, in whom the
qualities are not in equilibrium and which lead him towards one extreme, is not void of the others because of
that, but they do not exist in comparable proportion. He
carries the classification of the dominant one: he is said to
be of a temperament of fire, earth, water or air. Behold
medical nomenclature! Thus, I have given the nine temperaments and in that I make no innovations.

The temperaments of the seasons

What I am going to say about the seasons is only an
approximation for one cannot fix them with precise limits:
winter is inclined to the phlegmatic, spring stirs the blood,
yellow bile comes out in the summer, the black in the
autumn.

Classification of things which cause growth

We shall divide all things into mineral, vegetable and living animal possessing a body. It is the drug which conquers the illnesses of the body; it is the food which causes it to grow. The former also possesses a temperament; the latter is known by the taste; this opinion is accurate and true. Sweet, salty and bitter are the qualities of dryness; pungent of warmth; every tart, sour and astringent flavor extols dryness and cold. Everything which is aqueous and tasteless is balanced; everything which is fat is warm and moist; cold and moist are that which is tasteless and unpleasant.

On temperaments according to age

Every living being varies in temperament according to his age; but we shall speak especially of man. The temperaments of children and of young people are warm and very much alike, with a little more dryness for the latter and a little more obvious moisture for the former. The mature man is cold just as is the agèd one and so on. For both of them, there is a little more dryness together with the crudeness of humors for the agèd one.

Masculine and feminine temperaments

For males, warmth and dryness; for females cold and moisture.

Temperament according to the general appearance

The prosperous and fleshy body is cold and moist. People with a lean and slender appearance show dryness. All those whose veins are apparent are warm and cold are those whose dispositions are the opposite. The balanced temperament possesses the average (III-4).

Signs of the temperament inferred from colors and first on that of the skin

Do not infer any conjecture from the color of the skin if it is influenced by the country. For the Zendj (III-5) the heat of the climate has modified the color of the body to the point that their skin is covered with black. The Slavs have become light to such a point that they are of a brilliant whiteness. If you determined the seven climates, you would know their different temperaments. The fourth climate (III-6) is balanced; the color of its inhabitants depends on their temperament. The yellow complexion is that of the bile; the dark brown one is that of atrabile; redness depends on the great quantity of blood; ivory white characterizes the phlegmatic. The white complexion mixed with red construes a well-balanced temperament.

On the color of hair

He who has white hair has a cold temperament; the hair of the warm temperament is black; he who is less cold will have tawny hair; he who is less warm will have reddish hair; the one with a balanced temperament has tawny hair mixed with red.

On the color of eyes

When the crystalline lens and aqueous humor are of small volume, clear and transparent, brilliant and, moreover, outstanding, the eye is blue; the opposite conditions make it black. If the luminous medium is subdued, sight is less keen; if it is copious, the eye is sharp.

Third natural component—Humors

The body is made up of humors of different colors and of different temperaments. They are phlegm, yellow bile, blood and black bile. Natural phlegm is tasteless and mixed with cold; there is a variety known under the name of glassy, thick and of a cold temperament; another is sweet which is not void of warmth; there is also one called salty which leans towards warmth and dryness; another is acid and is the coldest; it is found in the sick stomach. Yellow bile allows several shades: one is known under the name of smoky; another is like the verdigris and the leek, which is the healthiest; another is like egg yolk and is not unhealthy; still another is a reddish color and is found in the gall bladder. Warmth is attributed to all. It is likely that the seat of black bile is in the spleen. The origin of the blood is in the liver; the veins transport it throughout the entire body. There is also some blood in the heart; it has a warm, moist character. The nature of the blood is preplexing; otherwise, it is not normal. It results from the mixture and the combustion of other humors.

Fourth natural component—Organs

The essential organs of the body are four in number; the others are only ramifications of them. One of them is the liver: the nutrition of the body depends upon it. The heart itself gives life; without it, man would be a plant; it is the source of natural warmth which follows the two large arteries. The brain, by way of the spinal cord and some nerves, prevents the heart from catching fire. It is from the latter that the motor influx of the joints leaves. The testicles themselves are the organs of reproduction; through them, the species perpetuate themselves; their absence causes them to disappear. The skin, flesh, different kinds of glands are the agents of the functions of the body. The bones, membranes, ligaments are the supports and protection of it. So that form and constitution be perfected, there are auxiliary organs of the principle one. The fingernails are tools for the extremities; hair eliminates the residues and ornaments the body.

Fifth natural component—Inspirations

The natural spirit is formed from a perfect and unspotted vapor. The animal spirit which is found in the heart maintains life. The vital spirit has the brain for a *substratum* and matures in the meninges. These different varieties are perfected in the cerebral convolutions; that is, likewise, the seat of feeling and thought. Each one of these spirits has strictly its own properties.

Sixth natural component—Forces

There are seven forces in human nature, different in appearance: one acts on the seed without giving it form; another gives the body of the embryo its shape, its size and its organs; another is attractive and maturing; another restrains and expels; a fifth distributes to the parts of the body what they need for food; the vital force is duple; likewise, its action: one acts on the pulse through dilatation and constriction of the arteries; its sister governs the feelings which involve actions, love, hate, baseness or elevation of the soul.

On the properties of the Soul

There are nine properties in the soul. Five of them are related: hearing, sight, smell, taste, and touch in its entirety; one goes to the nerves (III-7) ; through it man moves his joints; another represents objects as seen in a mirror (III-8); another governs thought; the last, memory.

Seventh natural component—Actions

Conditioned by forces, actions are equal in number to the former. Each one of them bears the corresponding name: attraction, variation, reservation; example: there is, thus, one of swallowing and of appetite for attraction constitutes a simple action, conditioned by a single force. The desire for food itself comes from two actions: intricate feeling and attraction; the actions of feeling and repelling produce change.

On the necessary factors—Air

The sun influences the air: this is true for the seasons and for the phases of the moon. It acts on climates with which we have already dealt.

On the influences of the stars in conjunction with the sun on air

The atmosphere changes its condition under the influence of the stars at their rising and setting. When the sun draws near, it puts fire into the air, whence shooting stars. It is similarly true that after this star has disappeared, the atmosphere has already become cool. If stars of evil omen appear, they decree death for men. If, on the contrary, they are of good omen, they determine absolute health.

On the variations of the air according to the countries and mountains

If a town is built upon a mountain, it is cold because of this. In a flat, low area, it is warmer; facing the south, it is warmer when the wind blows from the south. When back to back with the mountains on the south side, the north wind will chill it. Facing the west, its air will be heavier; contrariwise, on the east, the air will be lighter.

On the variations of the air according to the seas and winds

The seas have an opposite influence. That is what scientists have reported. Winds modify the atmosphere just as do the phases of the moon. The south wind possesses warmth and moisture for which reason it spoils things easily. The north wind possesses coldness and dryness; it brings on a cough. The east wind possesses warmth and tenuity; the west wind, coldness and heaviness.

On the variations of air because of the vicinity of certain terrains

Each region is moist in which soil is wet and around which marshes are found. If there are fresh water lakes around the town, it is moist. On the contrary, the air is dry in the vicinity of rocks and salty terrains.

On the variations of the climate according to residence

The residence provided with numerous openings receives all winds; it is very cold in winter, very warm in summer. It is just the opposite for a subterranean residence.

Variations of temperament according to clothing

Warmth is in silk and cotton materials, coldness in glossy and flax clothing. Warmth is in clothing made of camel hair and wool, but they have a little dryness.

Temperament of odors and perfumes

Every aromatic plant and every flower possess a warm temperament with the exception of five of them: myrtle, willow, water-lily, rose and violet which spread a cool aroma. Warmth is in perfumes and sweet-scented woods with the exception of sandal and camphor woods.

Influence of colors upon vision

The best colors for the sight are black and green. White and brilliant yellow are bad for the eyes for they are dazzling.

Second necessary factor—Food and Beverage

Be aware that it is food which ought to cause growth. For adults, it replaces instantly that which, being dissolved in the body, would decrease in quantity. The most commendable is the one which forms a pure blood when being transformed; for example, a good loaf of semolina (III-9), the meat of young chickens. Likewise, the vegetable beet agrees with sick people. Among foods certain ones are thick; example: semolina and two-year-old lambs with flavorful meat. The fish caught in rocky waters is a thick food which agrees with people who have to work hard. Among foods, there are some which, by themselves unpleasant to taste, are useful such as mustard, onion and garlic. In reality, they generate yellow bile; they are sometimes used as medicine. There are some which produce black bile and may make certain people sick; for example, old goats, old bulls, bread made from wheat with its impurities; that is dangerous. There are also those which create phlegm; for example, large fish and milk.

Rules concerning the beverage—Water or Others

Fresh river waters preserve their original moisture. They cause the elimination of residues and carry nourishment within the vessels. The best is rain water for it contains nothing harmful. Among all waters certain ones have lost their primitive qualities and have assumed those of the substance which is mixed in it. Wine, date wine and milk nourish the body. There are some which lend their temperament to the body; for example, oxymel (III-10) when it is assimilated.

Third necessary factor—Sleep and Wakefulness

Sleep is the rest of the forces of the body, motor as well as sensory. In reality, it warms the interior, whence more complete digestion of food. However, if it is prolonged, unhealthy humors fill the interior of the head. It moistens the body, relaxes and destroys the warmth which enlivens it. The state of moderate wakefulness causes the senses to function; it makes them active; it gives energy in action and thus, rids the body of its residues; but if it is prolonged, it becomes a restlessness which generates affliction and sadness; in reality, it debilitates the soul and the body, alters the complexion and the colors, makes the eyes sunken, disturbs digestion, lessens judgment and is emaciating.

Fourth necessary factor—Movement and Rest

Among physical exercises, there are some moderate ones; it is to them that one ought to devote himself. They balance the body by expelling residues and impurities and are factors of good nutrition for adults and of happy growth for the young. Unmoderated exercise is an over-load, alters the forces of the soul, leads to lassitude, consumes natural warmth, empties the body of its moisture, weakens nerves through the violence of pain and causes the body to age before its time. There is no illusion about prolonged rest: no advantages in its excess; it fills up the body with noxious humors and it does not place it in a state from which to benefit from its nourishment.

Fifth necessary factor—Elimination and Obstruction

The body needs elimination for all of its organs and for the brain. Phlebotomy and drugs, taken in the spring, are very useful for people. The emetic ought to be administered in the summer and the black bile expelled in the autumn. Gargle and cleanse your teeth in order to have your dentition and palate clean. Provoke urines; otherwise, fear dropsy. Expel the menstrua under pain of putrefaction. Use the purgative because with that, you will avoid the colic. Make use of baths in order to carry away impurities. Do not be slothful to make the residues come out of the pores and to rid the body of its uncleanliness. Allow sexual relations for young people: through them they will avoid masturbation. On the other hand, forbid them for the weak, old and debilitated people. Promise gout and pains for those who cohabit after the meal. The abuse of intercourse weakens the body and gives as a reward all kinds of illnesses.

Sixth necessary factor—Sensations

Rage causes warmth; sometimes it brings on illnesses. Fright brings on cold; sometimes it is such that it causes death. A great joy makes the body prosperous. There are some noxious ones which generate too much obesity. Sadness may be fatal to the emaciated; it is useful for those who wish to lose weight.

On Things Which Deviate from the Normal State

First on illnesses which overcome organs composed of organized parts

There are illnesses affecting the organs of which certain parts are organized. Some supervene because of a warmth without humors, such as phthisis and consumption. Certain ones come from humors linked to warmth, such as putrid fever. There are also some cold illnesses which produce no pus; example: frostbite by snow or cold. Others with humors, such as hemiplegia with a great quantity of phlegm. There are some moist ones without humors; the body is weak with this type. Moist ones with humors, such as the swelling of the abdomen with dropsy. There are dry illnesses with pus coming from wastes, such as cancer and buboes; and also the dry without humors; example: spasms with contractures.

Physical alterations of organs

In an organism physical alterations exist. A kind of illness involving the volume of the organ; increased, for example, too large a head; decreased, for example, too little a stomach. In the case of malformation, you may see a head like a basket. Likewise, there may be an alteration of the curvature; example, the sole of the foot lifted up by the flesh. It may happen that something is found in the ducts; for example, obstruction of the kidney by stones. That an organ which ought to be rough is found to be smooth; for example, too moist a stomach and vice versa; for example, the throat if it dries up. There may be alteration in the number, for example, six or four fingers; sometimes two fingers are joined; sometimes the jaws articulate poorly.

On the break of continuity

It applies to simple or complex anatomical elements. An example of the complex is the dislocation of the arm or the amputation of the foot or hand. An example of the simple: for bones, it is the fracture; for the membranous tissues and the vessels, it is the rent; at the level of the flesh, contusion and if it continues, ulceration; at the level of the muscles, abraision; of the skin, excoriation.

On abnormal factors—Causes

The causes are divided into external—those which reach the surface of the body—for example, fire or snow, a blow suffered, a split made by jumping, and into internal —which are of different kinds—for example, decomposition which brings on the so-called putrid fever. There are also antecedent causes which correspond to every state of retention in the body.

On the displacement of humors

Among the causes of illness, one admits that the temperament of an organ may be altered by the overflow of humors in it. It is necessary to face the power of thrust of the humor, the weakness of the receiver, the quantity of that evil humor and also the calibre of the vessels, the weakness of nutrition. That suffices to explain everything. Then, you will see, if it is dominated by that humor, that the organ may change temperament towards its opposite.

Causes of illnesses because of warmth

Whatever causes warmth brings great torments to the human body. Warmth may be inherent; for example, in garlic (III-11) ; it may be real; for example, in warm wind. Among these causes are the torments of the soul, like anger, and the movements of the body, like fatigue. Decomposition, lack of nourishment and everything which closes the pores of the skin like cold air.

Causes of illnesses because of cold

Everything which brings cold to the organism may succeed in causing a break of continuity. There exists an inherent coldness; for example, in henbane (III-12) if it is absorbed and a real cold, such as that of snow. Great hunger weakens the vital breath as the lamp lacks oil. Eating to repletion, in an exaggerated manner, smothers warmth. Violent and prolonged movements expel the vital breath and the body becomes cold. Rest by itself cools the body in the same manner that smoke extinguishes the flame. Excess thickness of the body retains warmth, leading to its own extinction. The emaciated body becomes cold to the point that you believe it radiates its heat.

Causes of illnesses because of moisture

There are five kinds of moistures; they are described and counted. Lukewarm fresh water brings true moisture by aiding the body. Inherently, the use of milk, fish and fresh cheese brings the moist element as does the rest of the body with excessive eating and accumulation of humors.

Causes of illnesses because of dryness

There exist five causes of dryness understood by the mind and preceived by the senses. In reality, certain ones dry: the north wind, for example; others have an inherent dryness, such as mustard. Hunger consumes the moisture of the body and, likewise, all violent movements and disturbances and also excess elimination as in diarrhea.

Causes of physical alterations

The causes of the excess of volume of organs are the formative power and alimentation. The causes of atrophy of organs are the opposite of the aforementioned ones. The cause of alteration of forms are the following: a bad constitution of the uterus or the paucity of readiness of sperm, or difficult expulsion of the fetus, whence alteration of its form by torsion; sometimes, it is the wet nurse who does not know how to swaddle the infant or to nurse him or to put him to bed correctly, or feeds him too much; sometimes weaning will be imperfect; sometimes his weakness causes the infant left to himself to fall; then, he may break a leg or thigh; falling on his nose may leave it flattened; medicine can do nothing for it; if following a fracture one does not have the patience to wait for healing, consolidation will never be perfect; sometimes it is the too great abundance of humors, elephantiasis or the opposite in chronic phthisis, torsion of the mouth made by relaxing the nerves (III-13) or by their contracture which causes the head to lean to one side; scars of abscesses and ulceration sometimes change the external appearance.

Causes of the obliteration of ducts

I have thought at great length in order to summarize the different causes of the occlusion of ducts. They are the exaggeration of the force of retention and the weakness of that of expulsion. Cold closes the ducts; dryness does it just as strongly and so does ligation. An abscess may compromise them; likewise, torsion and also astringent medication. That may happen after scarring of a wound or by vegetation or by the growth of a fleshy tumor; likewise, an accumulation of humors, pus, blood, curdled milk or water; this also occurs with abscesses, worms, stones, dry stools and gases.

Causes of the opening of ducts

They are the exaggeration of the force of expulsion and the weakness of that of retention. Drugs which open are warm and moist.

Causes of illnesses by altering the number

Everything which increases the number of organs or limbs comes from the excess of materials. If the material is good, for example, one has an extra finger; if it is bad, it is, for example, a ranula. Whatever decreases the number comes from the opposite of what I have stated above.

Causes of roughness or of flexibility

Whatever causes moisture to disappear causes roughness, such as a humor, smoke, powder, astringent food and certain drugs; a viscous humor and everything which is fat produce flexibility.

Causes of reunion and separation

Elements which are normally separated may reunite; an example is the joining of a surface wound of a limb with the wound of a neighboring limb. That comes from the exaggeration of the force of mutation and of the weakness of that of formation. It is the break of continuity which separates that which ought to be united normally in form as well as in position. This is true for all organs; here are the causes of this mishap.

Causes of the break of continuity

This may be a burning, decaying, corrosive or penetrating humor, a weight which demolishes or destroys or a viscous humor which separates articulations, an unfortunate leap which fractures, a wounding stone which causes a fracture; there are also corrosive and destructive medications; the scalpel and the air which causes splitting (III-14) by expanding and fire which acts upon the skin.

On abnormal effects—Symptoms

Certain illnesses are recognized through what the body produces, by what supervenes in it, by what is expelled: sputum, stools, sweat, urine. A normal function may be disturbed in three different manners: weakness, complete arrest and alteration. Each one has its own explanation. Weakness of function; example, for sight it is the decrease in light perception; the arrest of that function is blindness; alteration of function consists in seeing that which does not exist. Judge all organ disturbances by analogy with this example.

On the varieties of symptoms obtained from the state of the body

Symptoms are obtained through the physical examination of the body at certain moments. There are some visible ones, such as jaundice and edema; there are some perceptible to the ear, such as the gurgling of the abdomen in dropsy; the foul odor strikes at the sense of smell; for example, that of purulent ulcers; there are some accessible to taste, such as the acidity of the mouth; touch recognizes certain ones: the firmness of cancer!

Symptoms obtained from the products eliminated from the body

Symptoms obtained from the products eliminated from the body are accessible to the five senses. Urine may be red or black. Sputum may be bloody or frothy. There are some which signify an expulsion: flatulence, sneezing, hiccoughs. Vomitus may be acid, bitter or astringent. If urine is fetid, that indicates an ulcer of the bladder. As for sweat, it may be cold, thin or viscous. These symptoms are signs of illness for the patient and also are indications for the physician. I have summarized them above and now am going to delve into the details.

On symptoms in general

Every symptom has a value in the past, present and for the future. Example of past symptoms: the moisture of perspiring. By itself one of these signs is inadequate and cannot sway our opinion. That which indicates something of the present and of the future is absolutely necessary and serves as a foundation for our medicine. Among the symptoms, there are generalized ones and localized ones. I shall speak of the latter further along in the section on "Practice."

On general signs of the present

Every general sign refers to noble organs: liver, brain and heart are undeniably the principle ones.

Signs obtained from the functions of the brain

The healthy mind possesses an accurate imagination, reasoning and memory; normal movement and feeling indicate the integrity of the brain; their alteration signifies its illness.

Signs obtained from the functions of the heart

When the heart functions well as regards its beating, it is the sign of good health; the abnormal pulse indicates its alteration. It specifies afflictions and illnesses because of different kinds of disturbances.

On the different kinds of pulse and first on its amplitude

The kinds are ten in number, enumerated only for skillful physicians: the first, by measuring its amplitude, indicates excess or equilibrium; the full one presents important proportions during the examination; it gives information about the power of the heart; the weak one is just the opposite as regards the force; there are a long and a short, a narrow and a full, a superficial and a deep.

On the frequency of the pulse

The frequency of the pulse is in harmony with different characteristics. There is a quick and rapid one which indicates power and warmth; there is a slow and relaxed one which indicates weakness and cold.

On the slowness of the pulse

Measurement of the interval between beatings determines several possible varieties. Constant, without stopping, indicates weakness and warmth; intermittent, on the other hand, indicates softness and cold.

On the strength of the pulse

Its strength allows the recognition of two varieties: a strong one which thumps and its opposite, weak, which beats lightly.

On the consistency of the artery

The artery may be hard which indicates dryness or rather flexible which characterizes moisture.

On the temperature of the artery

The temperature of the artery gives exact information about the temperament: a cold artery indicates a cold temperament and vice versa.

What the artery contains

The artery contains humors of which I shall speak. The full one indicates an excess of humors and it is just the opposite for the empty one.

On the periods of pulsation and rest

The artery presents periods of rest and pulsation; it is palpation which recognizes them. The well-balanced pulse is in harmony with the age, the seasons of the year and the country. That is the normal pulse. There are some which are not in harmony; these are abnormal pulses.

On the quantity of arteries

Two types of arteries: the one of which the functions are harmonious, judged by the pulse and its opposite; the one which is normal has a steady function, the other one does not.

On the number of pulsations of the artery

The frequency of arterial pulsations may vary considerably. There are arteries with variable pulsations which present with two appearances: one is regularly irregular and the other is not; the patient does not perceive them. The one which is regular presents an alternant variety of which I shall speak; it strikes forcefully and then becomes a weaker beat. There is another kind of irregularity, another called the mouse's tail (III-15). There may be a variation in the course, itself, of a single pulsation. It is the touch which gives information (III-16). There are pulses which have received a surname and others which have not; we shall speak of the former. There is one called interrupted, another sustained, another low, another elevated. There is one which beats two times, others still more often; that indicates tumors and deep abscesses. One is called vermiform, another saw-tooth; one tingling, another undulating; another is called quivering, another that of phthisis. Each kind of pulse fits into two categories of which each one has two opposed varieties (III-17). Among them there is a balanced one, which has an exact dimension, but certain exaggerated varieties deviate from it. One recognizes the balance of the pulse through that which does not cause it to sway from one side to the other; the change of the pulse from its usual state is in harmony with the change of temperament of the individual.

On the pulse in harmony with age, the country, season, temperament, general appearance and sex

Be aware that different pulses exist according to ages, seasons, regions, temperaments of individuals, men and women, and their complexion. Warmth causes a rapid pulse just as do youth and being a male, and also southern countries, weakness, pregnancy and summer. In the cold country, the pulse is slow; likewise, for old men and during the winter, and also for women, obese people with weak flesh and in the northern countries. Every state of dryness causes firmness of the pulse; every state of moisture, its softness. Every pulse of a balanced temperament is also that way and, likewise, that of the spring. In the country of the fourth climate (III-18), the pulse is balanced. The pulse of the child is rapid and soft; that of the adult is slow and firm; the pulse of the one whose body is loaded with humors is full; after evacuation, the pulse is empty and confined.

Signs obtained from expectoration

The chest and lungs are organs of respiration; if they are healthy, life is secure; if their function is abnormal, the heart becomes inflamed. It is expectoration which marks illness of the chest. An illness which has not yet matured has no expectoration; the appearance of maturation is shown by a very fluid expectoration. If it is average, that indicates that the illness is in the middle of its phase of ascension; very abundant and thick, that signifies the end of the development; fluid expectoration shows that the causal humor is itself acute which means that drainage will be rapid. It is just the opposite if it is thick; black sputum marks the violence of inflammation; green sputum, a porraceous bile; that with a bright yellow tinge, an egg-yellow bile. White indicates phlegm; the red, blood. Fetid sputum proves decomposition within the lung; the absence of offensiveness removes that idea. If the sputum has a round form and if the patient is febrile, realize that there is an effusion. If there is no fever, one is dealing with phthisis. Mature sputum is rejected without cough, and is white, thick, homogeneous and without odor in the beginning.

Symptoms obtained from the function of the liver

It is in the liver that the humors are born; from there they are spread throughout the body. Every organ functions because of it and it alone has no need of the others. The vital spirit is born in the vapor of the liver; the body is healthy according to its state. If the humors are healthy, the body is; the former are if the liver is in good state. Water carries food to it and the water is mixed with the predominant humor and, with its expulsion in the urine, shows that it contained residues. Urine has different colors and everything that the humors have left in it appears to us as a sediment. It is apparent, from what I have stated and wise men witness it, that urine is a faithful guide for the knowledge of the illness.

On urine and first about the color

While urine witnesses the quantity of ingested food and drink, it is a sign of bad digestion, phlegm, cold, restlessness or of hepatic obstruction. Somewhat yellow, it indicates the presence of a certain quantity of bile. The color of fire, that means the presence of a great deal of yellow bile. Very yellow and tinted with red, it proves a super abundance of yellow bile. Dark red urine of the one who has not ingested saffron (III-19) and who has had neither fever nor colic contains blood. When found black after having been dark, it signifies that the patient has suffered a great chill. Black after having been very red indicates a poor combustion of humors. Judge the illness according to the odor of urine on the condition that the patient has not ingested a coloring food, certain vegetables, cassia fistula (III-20) and that which may tint like murri (III-21).

On the density of urine

The tenuity of the urine indicates inadequacy of digestion. Sometimes it is fluid after indigestion or obstruction of the liver or because of a tumor. The thickness of the urine indicates good digestion or the abundance of phlegm in the body.

On the sediments in urine

The white sediment indicates recovery; yellow, it marks acuteness of the bile; if it is red like the bloodwort (III-22), it is a question of disease of the blood. If a similar sediment continues without modification, that indicates an abscess of the liver. Black after having been dark red and that after loss of strength, going to the bottom after having floated, that means the soul is about to escape; the patient can no longer benefit from the prayers of a sorcerer; death is at hand through the excess of humoral combustion. If the sediment appears black after having been dark and if it does not occur in the course of an acute illness, especially if this appearance coincides with a favorable sign, and if the origin of the illness is in black bile, it indicates the end of the illness.

On the location of the sediment

If a cloud appears floating in the upper portion of the vial, it indicates crudeness of the illness. If a certain maturity exists in the urine, wind (III-23) is causing the sediment to reascend to the surface. If the sediment is half-way up, be aware that the wind is in a small quantity. If it is white, after having been yellow, coherent without being thick, falls to the bottom, appears with a changeable color (III-24), it marks the maturity of the illness.

On the consistency of the sediment

An ephemeral sediment indicates the weakness of the patient. If there are elements similar to barley meal in the urine, one is dealing with scrapings of the vessels (III-25). If the sediment looks like bran and has a bad odor, it indicates ulceration within the ducts; like metal filings, it proves the elimination of portions of organs. If pus appears in the vial, it marks the opening of a collection. If the sediment has decomposed blood, there is a phlegmonous tumor. If it goes to the bottom, resembles sperm, it comes from an immature lymph swelling. If one sees sand in it, be aware that there is a calculus.

On the odor of urine

If the urine has no odor, it is that the food has not been digested or has been ingested raw. The degree of decomposition agrees with the intensity of the odor of the urine. If this odor is dreadful, be aware that the illness is in the bladder. Thus, I have reported on the different kinds of urine; guide yourself by what I have stated about their composition.

Signs obtained from the examination of stools—on their quantity

The stools give information about the state of the stomach, sometimes about the intestine and the liver. If they are sparce, it is that nourishment has been carried toward the organs, or that the repelling force is weak, the drawing force strong because of an illness and that indicates that the body of the patient is full of noxious residues. But if they are abundant, they indicate that the food has done no good or that the power of assimilation is weak and the expelling force is weak because of an illness. If they are white, there is an obstruction of the biliary tracts or a tumor; jaundice is the visible witness, the urine equally yellow; or the body is in a very bad state following an illness due to phlegm or too cold a temperament. If the stools are red or fire colored, that indicates an excess of yellow bile. If they are porraceous or verdigris, there is a developing illness. Black, they show evidence of a chronic and violent chill within the body of the patient and if that is produced during an acute illness, death is at hand. Hard stools show the power of the force of assimilation, a burning heat or a constringent food. Soft and light, they mark the paucity of the force of assimilation, there is coldness within the body which is changing it or the food was a laxative. If the stools are delayed, it is a sign of digestion difficulty at the level of the intestines, weakness of the force of expulsion, of coldness or that the intestines are retaining them. Expelled rapidly, they prove that the food is slippery and does not linger, that the moisture of the humors is cast into the stools abundantly, that the mesentery has no drawing force or that the intestine is affected; one may be dealing with ulcers, indigestion or even another illness. If they are expelled with noise, that means an excess of intestinal gas. If they contain pus, that marks intestinal tumors. If there is blood with expulsion, that means excoriation (III-26). If they are fetid, there is a serious putrefaction. If they seem to be coated with oil, that indicates liquefaction of the body fat. Their sour-wine odor means acid phlegm.

Signs obtained from sweat

An abundant sweat is a symptom of moist illnesses. It is a sign of a strong temperament; that is not true of intermittent sweating. A very abundant perspiration coinciding with a progressive weakening of the patient means the diminution of strength of his being and his death is at hand. In the course of illnesses, a light perspiration indicates closure of the pores, thickness of the humors, debility of the expulsive force, lack of maturation of food and softness of the body of the patient.

Meaning of perspiration

If in the course of an illness sweat is white, this illness is phlegmatic; yellow, for yellow bile; black, for atrabile; red, it indicates an illness of the blood; its flavor may also be a guide. A thin perspiration means thinness of the humors; similarly, its thickness. If it affects the whole body, it is a good sign; localized, it is troublesome. If it appears at an opportune time or at a period of crisis, it is an excellent and commendable sign; in the opposite case, it is far from being good.

On prognosis—general signs

There are those which correspond to a serious illness capable of attacking a healthy man and others which give information about an illness in the course of its development. The guides of the first case are the following: abundance or diminution (III-27) in all parts of the body and brain. Abundance of these humors indicates the customs of rest and of copious alimentation. The scarcity of warm baths and of physical exercise brings on illnesses by plethora. The opposite allows one to fear illness related to inanition.

Signs of plethora and first—its harmony with the force of the individual

The kinds of plethora are in harmony with the forces of the man. If it attacks the force which changes, the patient has no appetite; in the urine, no visible sign of maturity, soft stools. If it touches the force of movements, you will see them difficult. If it is in harmony with the pulsation force, you will find pulsations weak; the cause of weakening of these forces is in the intolerance in juxtaposition with chyme of which too small a quantity does not succeed in filling the cavities.

On plethora within cavities (III-28)

Another kind of plethora is that of hollow organs on the condition that their content be fluid. This fluid may be unspotted blood, bile or phlegm. Sometimes the souls have a flourishing health and the chyme does not make them heavy.

Signs of the predominance of the blood

If among the humors the blood carries predominance, sleep and migraine are exaggerated, vessels turgid and red, sometimes thought revolts; there is a heaviness of the head, weakness of sensation, carelessness, warmth to the touch, heaviness of the shoulders, yawning; sometimes heaviness of the flanks; nose bleeding, the desire to stretch out, relaxing of the abdomen, search for a life of well-being, dreams, varied joys, and of all colors, gaiety, longings for phlebotomy, unusual ruddiness of the eyes, furuncles and pustules, dreams of sweet things, a sugar flavor in the mouth, as if the patient had just eaten some, appear. If these symptoms are seen in the spring or during the prime of youth, they indicate diseases of the blood. I shall deal with this in the "Practice" portion.

Signs of the predominance of the bile

If bile is predominant, the shade of the body is yellow, the appetite weak, the mouth bitter. There are gastric burning, vomiting of bile, a powerful diarrhea, restlessness, sunken eyes, dry mouth and tongue. Between times the urine is yellow, the patient has episodes of syncope, some goose-bumps, is sad, is thirsty without appetite and dreams of flames; his pulse is weak, his body febrile. Frequent warm baths are the cause of this state as are sojourns in southern countries, youth and the prolonged misuse of spiced foods, especially in the summer.

Signs of the predominance of the black bile

If black bile predominates, the body is wan, thoughts sullen, appetite reduced, an acid flavor in the mouth. On examination, anguish, rigidness of the face, pulse firm in its slowness; the patient is constipated, presents black spots, sadness, restlessness without agitation. Urines are white, not very dense, crude; similarly, the stools are not digested. The causes are dry food, anxiety, permanent sadness and misery. In his dreams, the patient sees dangers and completely frightening things. This affects the mature age in autumn, in northern countries and the weakened man.

Signs of the predominance of phlegm

If phlegm predominates, the head is heavy, the sleep prolonged; there is a laziness of movements, little appetite; plethora is in harmony with the force of the individual; he is slow in his gait, his intelligence is slow, he leans towards an unusual softness, foams, has a swollen face, his shade is dull; the pulse is slow and thick; urine dense, strong and crude; thirst is reduced except when the phlegm is salty or decayed. The cause of this state is cold and moist food, old age, winter, sedentarity, lack of warm baths, sometimes gluttony, the sojourn in a country damp because of its water flow; in his sleep, the phlegmatic person dreams of seas, complains of nightmares and his chyme is not digested well. If you see these exact symptoms, messengers of illness in individuals in good health, endeavor to make them disappear.

On prognostic signs in the course of illnesses

There are those which warn about death and others which indicate healing. We shall give a description of some which will allow them to be known. The physician will be the judge of these signs because of his science; he will know if the patient ought to die and will forego treating him; likewise, he will know if he can cure and will announce it. It is necessary for him to recognize from the very first the periods of illness and their complications, their duration, long or short, their seriousness or their benignancy; he ought to strive to know the accidents which may supervene in the different periods and to foresee the crisis.

On the knowledge of periods in the course of illnesses

Every illness possesses periods ending in death or healing. There is a period of beginning, one of ascension, a state in which death is possible, a fourth, subsidence, in which there is no risk of death except for mistakes. The beginning is the period of functional disturbances and of weakness of organs in their performance; it is so true that you will verify the disturbance of digestion in the excreted residues: sputum, stools, urine. You will recognize the period of ascension by the duration of attacks of fever and by associated symptoms (III-29). The period of the state which follows it is characterized by complete maturity: febrile attacks no longer increase; the symptoms become stabilized. Then, the illness begins to decrease: the fourth period. Sometimes it ends in a beneficial crisis. If you see this sign, inform the patient of his cure. Death does not supervene during the period of subsidence if there has not been a mistake in the treatment or if an illness mixed with the atmosphere (III-30) does not supervene or any other attacking him on the surface. Our knowledge of the beginning of the illness will lead us to prescribe a light diet; in the period of ascension it will be necessary to maintain a proper internal medium: that is an aid to one's lucky star; when the end of the illness has come, be very cautious with the dietary regimen.

On the duration of illnesses

Every illness has its duration: the short one is called acute; it kills in a short while or ends with a favorable crisis; it matures rapidly; its periods are very close together and teeming in accidents. You will recognize it by the abruptness of its beginning. Then, allow your patient an accommodating diet; do not give him too much nourishment for his strength nor any too small and unsubstantial; otherwise, you will change everything from the beginning and it will not come to an end. On the other hand, let the food be measured wisely for him like provisions for a traveler. If you see any danger signals appear, of malignancy or pain, if the strength of the patient declines, if his reasoning is disturbed, if he raves, if he does not sustain his illness, warn him of his probable death before the end of the development. Be aware that death is foreseen by grievous signs and by bilious manifestations. There exist illnesses of long duration, called chronic, which only change the organism slowly but which kill by consumption, phthisis, hemorrhage, anemia; they may heal after a long development and end by maturity and dissolution. You will recognize them by the lack of the seriousness of symptoms and by the fact that they are cold; do not feed

your patient inadequately: he will lose strength. Between
these two kinds of illnesses, there is one of intermediate
duration, neither short nor long, for which the diet should
be medium in strength and amount.

On the signs of the crisis

Be aware that the crisis is a brutal and rapid change
which is produced in the course of acute illnesses and
means the battle between the latter and the patient. It re-
solves in a short while, be it death or be it healing. Between the strength of the patient and the illness exists
such a violent hostility that it is a veritable war; if the
strength has it, the crisis is favorable whence survival and
safety; if the illness has the victory, it means death.

On the different aspects of the crisis

There exist six aspects in the development of the
crisis: a slow, a rapid; in a short while the individual
passes to the best and to the cure; this favorable solution
is preceded by good signs—that is the pre-eminently for-
tunate crisis. There is another rapid change which leads
to a fatal outcome. The fourth is a slow evolution which
leads the patient to a dangerous door (III-31). It is not
only that strength is dissolved but rather the consumption
of the organism. The fifth is intermediate between the
fatal developments. The sixth leads to healing in a short
while. These last two aspects of the crisis are called complex; they oppose each other. The favorable crisis supervenes after complete maturity of the illness with preservation of all the strength of the patient. The opposite supervenes during the ascension of the illness; it is troublesome.

On the signs to know pertinent to the crisis

There are three things to know pertinent to the crisis:
the messenger signs, the critical days and their favorable

or fatal meaning. That will inform you about the outcome
of any crisis.

On the messenger signs of the crisis

Every crisis is indicated by the violence of the following
symptoms: mental and sensory troubles, pain in the ears or
head, flow of tears, agitation, loss of sleep, motor difficulties, restlessness, thoracic or cervical pain, anguished awak-
ening, disturbed and red eye, grinding and chattering of
teeth, itching of the nose, turned up or sucking lips, rapid
respiration, a thirst for fresh air with agitation, permanent rapidity of the pulse, frequent cough with rumbling
of the throat, permanent palpitations of the heart with
syncope, involuntary rising and walking, pain in the throat
with pharyngeal constriction and following that, prolonged
syncope, tingling in the bowels and sides with painful
paroxysms, permanent uneasiness of the stomach. Sometimes the patient complains about his spleen or his liver,
endures abdominal, pubic, renal and bladder difficulties,
experiences violent pains in the pelvis, penis or uterus,
suffers with joint pain or only with certain ones on the
outside as well as inside. If you see these signs increase
during the critical days, it is favorable and especially if
the illness is mature; otherwise, the meaning is the opposite.

On the days of crisis

The cause of the crisis, if what they say is true, is the
influence of the moon on illnesses; it is, in reality, a star
with rapid movements, making its revolution in a short
time, possessing a period of waxing and one of waning and
that is well-known by astronomers. Its influence is not
perceptible by the senses, whether of good or evil omen,
whereas her quarters are visible because of the illumina-
tion of the sun. The quarter moon governs the four day

intervals and when half full, the seven day intervals. The illness which begins when the moon is in conjunction with stars of evil omen (III-32) is fatal. If it remains when the moon is in conjunction with stars of good omen (III-33), the patient survives and his days are prolonged. If it continues during the moon's conjunction with the ones of evil omen, the patient dies, his life is drained and he disappears. Crises supervene most often on the quarternary days, sometimes on the septenary days. In this case, it is excellent and is accompanied by messenger signs of good omen; the maturity is its witness. These quarternaries and septenaries are exact periods; without them, there is no fixed duration for a reason hidden by Allah. Oh, but that is difficult! The illnesses which have neither maturity nor messenger signs are, on the other hand, dangerous; they have no crisis and if they do, it is a sign of fatal relapse.

Signs indicating the end of the crisis

If you see a tenacious, serious illness of the blood show troublesome symptoms with cerebral accidents afterwards affecting all the senses, if blushing and nasal pruritus appear, the end of the crisis will be marked by a nose bleed. If accidents occur on the lower part of the body, continuous pains around the umbilicus, retention of the menstrual flow, the end will be the appearance of menstruation. If there are no pains of the upper portion of the body but under the sides, if the patient complains of his liver and the pain radiates towards the anus, you will make no error by announcing healing after a hemorrhoidal flow. If the illness comes from yellow bile and during the period of decline a swelling of the head appears, migraine with pains, do not be impatient: the crisis will end with a nose bleed. If mishaps lie at the level of the stomach of a patient who suffers with his liver, with nausea and syncope, the crisis will end with vomiting. If there is no headache but the patient suffers with his abdomen, with swelling of the umbilicus and if there is constipation, be on guard: the crisis will end with an intestinal flow. If there are no colic, no serious symptoms, few disturbances, no restlessness, no perspiration, if the illness develops without acuity, with suprapubic pains, remember from me this precise opinion: the crisis will be urinary. If the patient urinates without retention, does not complain about his pubis, if the pores of his skin are open and if there are no violent pains, nor dryness, nor restlessness, the crisis will be manifested by sweating. If there are pains at the crossroads of lymph nodes, the crisis will occur with their suppuration. Treat your patient with the conduct inspired by the signs indicating death or survival.

On the messenger signs of death and first on those based on the actions of the patient

Among these are fear of light, flowing of tears with a lot of blinking of the eyelids, diminution in the opening of the eye on one side, deviation of the gaze, opening of the mouth without yawning, permanent position of the neck, flaccidity of hands and feet. If the patient leaves his bed, if he uncovers his feet and hands, assumes a bad appearance, begins to pull the threads of his clothes, if his extremities are heavy, his gaze fixed, if there are abnormal grindings of the teeth, groping of the hands about the pillow, if he sees a young man in black wanting to kill him, and that during an acute illness, death is at hand. If our patient, usually taciturn, begins to talk idly, if our usually calm one shows impatience, complains of no longer seeing or hearing, or if he has completely lost his strength, if, at the end of his sleep, he sees himself covered with snow, if he is agitated and experiences a great chill, that is a fatal sign. If there are nocturnal restlessness, loss of sleep or sleeping during the day or if when sleep returns, the condition does not improve, the sickness is serious. It is, likewise, a bad sign if there is no improvement after treatment done according to the rules (III-34).

On the messenger signs of death obtained from the condition of the body

If the face becomes like that of a dead man, hair glued to the temples by the illness, if the ears are twisted by the cold, the eyes irritated and hollowed, red or black, outstanding or if a tarnished color, glassy, motionless and fixed, cold or if the eyelids are inverted, if the nose is pointed, leans to one side, if one side of the lip is turned up, if the extremities are cold, if an ulcer and some black elements appear on the tongue, all that joined with impatience and agitation is a sign of death during an acute illness. If there is a bluish or green shade of the nails with the appearance of black spots on the body, if jaundice appears before the seventh day with depression of the hypochondria, if the body is cold on the surface and warm inside, and especially if this is manifested at the level of the principle organs, if edema of the face and extremities appears before the end of the second septenary, it is an adequate sign that the patient will not see the end of this septenary; likewise, if fever disappears without crisis or if you see it intensify on two consecutive days.

Signs of approaching death obtained from waste materials

Black stools, green, red, offensive and greasy, watery or buttery, white—all that is troublesome. Stools which are of different colors announce death in the absence of a crisis. If you see the patient lacking appetite in the course of a frankly bilious affliction, if he excretes a few clots of black blood and then some scrapings of flesh, all that after bilious stools and without burning pain, if black stools appear after a period of abnormal weakness, this is a bad sign. If there is constipation in the course of an acute fever, that affects the brain. For a cautious man, the act of releasing noisy flatus contrary to his custom is a bad sign. Thin, black urine, decreased in amount, is a sign of death. Delirium with diminution of urine is the worst of misfortunes. Vomiting, draining of the black and putrid blood through the nose indicates decomposition of the body. Frequent cough with little expectoration in the case of phthisis is a bad sign. Difficult expectoration of different colors with coughing indicates an approaching death. Sweating of the brain followed by eliminations which do not relieve the patient is a bad sign.

Messenger signs of healing

If the facies of the patient appear similar to when he was in good health, the cure is at hand. If a balanced warmth appears and the hypochondria are not shrunken, if, after the seventh day, a jaundice appears and the mind is healthy, there is no danger. The acuity of the senses, the strength of movements, the lightness of the limbs are a good sign. If he sleeps at night as usual and not during the greater portion of the day, if he is quiet after a sleep which has dissipated his pains, his delirium and has rested him from his illness, it is favorable. In the case of an affliction of the brain and its related organs during the illness, if there is no longer any permanent delirium, the patient will be easily saved. If sneezing appears during a delirium, it is a sign of healing; likewise, epistaxis or otorrhagia during an illness of the head. A regular respiration, neither rapid nor slow, is one of the best signs; there are no good signs in the case of irregularity nor when the patient stands erect to breathe noisily. It is favorable when the pulse is full, not restrained and when the breath of the patient is not burning. Among the good signs, the favorable consistency of normal stools and of a yellow color, neither dark black nor green, it is a symptom of survival if on the day of crisis one finds worms; the stools excreted thusly carry the illness with them. If the patient expels bile, deafness disappears and so do the pains in a case of a cerebral illness. The blood of hemorrhoids comes from the spleen and from black bile; its drainage cures them. The excretion of water and of phlegm cures dropsy. The expulsion of yellow bile accelerates the cure of ophthalmia. If you see lemon colored urine with a white sediment at the bottom of the container, if, during a continuous fever, you verify a moderate sweating, if the neck glands swell exteriorly during a sorethroat, it is a good sign. During a chronic cough, testicular swelling is a sign of healing; likewise, that of a foot or of a crural region during illness of the lung. Herpetic ulceration of the nostrils or of a lip during intermittent fever announces healing. The appearance of varices cures alopecia and also afflictions of the abdomen and of the spleen. Sour discharges during lientery (III-35) come from the retention of food. Fever supervening during spasms or epilepsy announces healing. The hiccough heals through eructation.

On the ways to establish a prognosis according to the symptoms

When you wish to judge the condition of a patient, weigh the different symptoms. There are some which indicate a good state of strength; others contradict it. Give a certain value to those obtained from the examination of

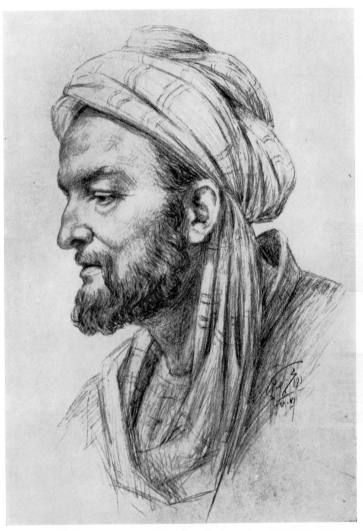

A frequently encountered painting of Avicenna.

the brain. You will see no sign of certainty occur in the same patient with opposing conditions. When the symptoms are contradictory in a weak patient, their value is not great. If only troublesome signs exist, that means death. If light symptoms are contradictory, doubt persists, reserve your judgment and wait to commit yourself. If the signs are balanced, wait longer and judge according to the dominant ones when the balance sways.

SECOND PART
Practice and Its Divisions

Thus, I have expounded upon what you have just read in verse in the portion on Theory. Such was my intention. Here I am beginning the account of Practice. I announced at the beginning of my work what it will be necessary to state in this discourse. Practice comprises two sections: one is carried out with the aid of hands; the other with drugs and a suitable dietary regimen. In reality, what one can obtain from a diet is not to be scorned. This includes two kinds: one, a preserver of health; the other one, curing the illness, and that, during my lifetime, is the physicians' aim.

MEDICAL PRACTICE
Chapter I
On the Conservation of Health Through Diets and Drugs

The preservation of health can be extended to such persons who are completely healthy. For the one with imperfect health, there are two cases to face: the one is that in which the patient is afflicted throughout his whole organism at all times, such as the old man, the convalescent, the young infant, and the one in whom you discover signs causing a fear of the illness. The other is the one of the patient whose affliction is localized in the skin, the flesh or the bones. Example: the one whose stomach is naturally weak and cold, the one who suffers with her uterus, the one who has a sixth digit or a tumor, the one who is ill at a certain age or at a certain time of the year, like the one who is weak in his youth and strong in adulthood or another one, with a dry temperament, who becomes weak in autumn and gets along well in the spring.

Hygiene of the healthy man in harmony with the atmosphere, particularly in summer

To preserve health, there are two practices in medicine. If you have to maintain the temperament of someone in good condition, give him a suitable diet. If you decide to transform an organism from his natural state, give him that which is contrary to his temperament. Regarding this healthy man, control him, in general, in a way to maintain him in this good condition. Advise him to live in countries of the fourth climate (III-36), those in which the air is healthy, a place above the desert, facing the east; the air is lighter there. For the summer, choose mountains and countries open to the north. For the night, occupy the upper floors and during the day, the lower floors. Avoid wool and cotton clothes, choose light flax, use cold aromatic substances such as rose oil; protect your eyes from the dust, keep from breathing smoke, the unhealthy vapors, avoid the sun's direct rays, the simoon (III-37), and the intense heat of the day. Do not read fine letters very long, nor small inscriptions nor difficult writings.

On the dietary regimen in general

It is proper to eat at least once in the space of a day and night, at most twice, the average being three times in two days. It is necessary to chew well to obtain good digestion; everything which is hard to chew is hard to digest. When you eat an indigestible food, wisely take something to neutralize it, its opposite, considering its temperament. In reality, there exist some poorly balanced temperaments which an abnormal food suits. In this case, habit becomes a force. Satisfy your desire. Suppress a detrimental habit only gradually. Prefer moist meals, dispel the astringent ones, mix acid with the agreeable sweet flavor. Improve whatever is dry with the moist, whatever is cold by the warm; if the meat is warm, mix it with a cold one; if it is moist, mix it with its opposite; if you fear the unhealthfulness of fat and its difficult digestion, add some salt or acid to it—both will make it digestible.

The hour of the meal

It is following exercise and after having defecated that it is proper to eat. Benefit from a moment of leisure; look for a fresh and ventilated place, a cool hour; be cautious about this matter.

Dietary regimen in summer

In the summer, reduce the amount of food and look for light nourishment; avoid all heavy meat; prefer vegetables and milk foods, fresh fish, young goats and lambs, chickens, hens, partridge and francolin (III-38) flesh, all meat seasoned with coriander, in the form of a stew, with sourgrape sauce and zirabaj (III-39), avoid sweet foods like habis (III-40), leek omelettes (III-41), egg white;

prefer hulame (III-42), qaris (III-43); eat tifsil (III-44) and masus (III-45).

On the beverage

If you wish to avoid illness, divide your nourishment into three parts: a third for respiration, a third for food and the rest for water. A little cold water quenches thirst, better than far too much warm water. Too much ice in the beverage is harmful to the nerves; allow it only for the obese and sanguine man with strong tissues. It is not necessary to drink at the table except with the threat of choking and never after the meal, nor after a warm bath, nor after a violent exercise, nor after sexual intercourse— that can be dangerous. If it is necessary and you can control yourself, drink moderately. When digestion is completed in the lower part of the stomach, then have the amount of water which quenches your thirst and a sufficiency of wine. But after having quenched your thirst with water and wine, if you are thirsty again, drink no more— that thirst is false.

On fermented beverages

As regards drinking, do not misuse wine. Be content with a small amount and, then, not every day, nor with fasting, nor after a light or acid food. Do not get intoxicated incessantly. If that happens to you, let it be only once a month. Wine taken in small quantities is useful; in large amounts it is dangerous. Warm and intoxicate the one who stuns easily; give him aromatics and let him eat sour pomegranates, quince, cucumbers at the same time; dilute his wine with water. Give it straight to the one in whom it provokes flatus. The best wine is the strong yellow kind; it is proper to drink it with salty meats. During the summer, it is better to drink a light and thin white wine; mix it with water, eat acid meats and, then, eat astringent meats.

On sleep

Do not sleep too long—it is detrimental for the mind! Do not stay awake too long for your senses will be weakened. It is proper to prolong sleep after a meal difficult to digest or after one of indigestion. Do not sleep too much when you are hungry—the vapors springing forth from the humors will ascend to the brain. After the meal, sleep with the head elevated so that your food will take its proper place of digestion.

On physical exercise

Do not give up hard exercise; do not seek rest too long; preserve a happy medium. Exercise your limbs to help them repel the bad humors by walking and struggling until you succeed in panting. The thin man ought to avoid exercises in order not to increase his exhaustion. Do just the opposite for the fat man and make him wear a girdle if he has a fat abdomen. In summer, decrease fatigue for perspiration is exhaustion. I have reported in the theoretical part on the diet which agrees with the body to expel residues, to retain that which ought to be and to deal with the disturbances of the soul.

Another dietary regimen according to the seasons

Remember all that I have said concerning the summer diet and its use for fiery temperaments, young people and in southern countries. During the winter, do just the opposite to fight against the severity of the cold. In spring and autumn, follow a plan half-way between the winter and summer. In spring, use a diet less dry than in winter. In autumn a more moist one; avoid dryness. Use a summer diet for the end of spring and the beginning of autumn. The beginning of spring is like the end of autumn. Feed them, as in winter, with warming-up meats. The above diets are valid for sedentary life; for the traveler use the facts below.

Hygiene of the traveler and especially on the sea

For those who travel on land and sea, avoid sea voyages in winter and land voyages during the rainy season. Whoever travels by sea ought to carry enough water and be provided with a good cistern. For his voyage, give him moist and laxative food; if he fears seasickness, purge him and administer to him acid syrups mixed with some astringent liquids. To avoid uncleanliness, obtain changes of clothes for him. In the course of the trip, if lice multiply and he cannot get rid of them, it is necessary for him to take some wool, make a ribbon with it, dip it in mercury, rub himself with it, and wear this ribbon around his neck among his clothing until the real destruction of the lice. Proceed as you would in cold weather for the one who travels on land.

Hygiene of the traveler on land and particularly in the cold season

Warn him about the snow to avoid frostbite. Satisfy him so that he does not die from hunger. If he is attacked by chilling, give him a warm bath and place him with florid people. If the frost dims his vision, cover him with a black veil. Have him carry black in his hands and let him look at it for a long time. Protect extremities from the cold by wrapping them with costus oil (III-46). Let his feet be bound for a long while before placing them in his shoes. If, following frostbite, the patient suffers no longer with his feet, it is that the cold has dealt them a blow. Then, untie the bindings, rub and warm him. For that use warm mustard oil; then cover and protect them. If they have become black, carry out scarifications below the black part; if decay appears in it, clean them. If the decomposed portion breaks away, cut it off; I mean, cut off that decayed portion. Treat the one who is tired with oil rubs; give him rich food; place him in a warm bath, washing the entire body and let him remain at rest for several days.

Hygiene of the traveler during warm weather

Attend him on his departure and return. Prevent him from traveling when the hot wind blows to avoid heat stroke. Draw some blood from him, an amount of some consequence. Thus, he will avoid any risk of sickness. It is necessary to purge the man with copious bile if you fear his thirsting; destroy it with syrups before his departure for the heat is dangerous; feed him lightly with cool vegetables; let him drink a large amount of water all at once, rest as long as possible without becoming unnerved, use parasols, cover his head, not cry out and not talk too much; let him not debate nor contend nor expose himself too long to the heat of the sun. If you are very thirsty while traveling, keep some pills of camphor of the size of a small lupine (III-47). Drink some purslane juice (III-48) and some sourgrape juice diluted with water. If you fear a change in your complexion because of the sun because it disfigures you with spots, use oil mixed with wax as one does in the harems.

On the subject of infants still within the bosom of their mother

It is proper to protect the infant within the maternal bosom so that nothing disturbing attacks him. Take precautions as regards the food of the pregnant woman so that her taste does not become depraved. It is necessary to improve her blood and that her residues be expelled for it is from her blood that the infant is formed. If the blood of the pregnant woman is agitated, do not bleed her; cool her and extinguish her burning. If she carries a disturbed humor, do not purge her; quiet the violence.

Management of the delivery

When the time of delivery arrives, it is necessary to use that which may facilitate it. In a warm bath rub the hips of the parturient and the neighboring regions of her genital parts with oil so that the nerves relax and so that there will be no fatigue at the time of delivery. Let her food be mostly fat; make her drink greasy broth. Protect her from noise, jumping, terrors, clamoring and trauma. If the delivery is difficult, let her take a decoction of dates and fenugrec (III-49) ; choose for her an intelligent midwife who will stretch out the former's legs without pity and, then, will make her sit down in a single blow while pressing skillfully over her abdomen. In case of a serious loss of blood, give her some yellow amber (III-50) pills; if the flow of blood is too weak, use pills of aloes (III-51) . If the after-birth (III-52) does not come down, fumigate with dissolving agents such as aloes, tar, savin (III-53) , sulfur (III-54) and colocynth (III-55) .

On the choice of a wet-nurse

If the child is to be fed by a wet-nurse, intrust him with only one of a certain age (III-56) . Choose a wet-nurse of an average age, fleshy, with tight skin, of a well-balanced temperament, with a firm body, with voluminous breasts, whose head and eyes are clean, who has no internal illness, whose limbs and joints are robust, whose milk is neither too liquid nor too thick, white in color, sweet and pleasant to taste, with a good odor and homogeneous when one expresses it. Give her a sweet and fatty diet, fresh fish prepared in oil.

Special hygiene of the infant

Before swaddling him, rub him with astringents until his skin is toughened; then, wash him in warm water to rid him of his impurities and squeeze him gently. Do not keep him too long at the breast to avoid indigestion; do not deprive him of eating too long to dispel fever. Do nothing which may upset him, prevent or disturb his sleep. For sleeping, place him on a soft bed in a dark spot; add a little poppy (III-57) to his food if illness prevents his sleeping. When awake, let him see the light, the sky and its stars. During the day, have the colors vary before him to train his sight; speak to him in a loud voice to accustom him to the spoken word; let him suck on honey; put some on his palate and tongue; to this honey add a little liquorice and incense syrup and leave it in his mouth. Give him some nasal instillations for relief or cleaning purposes; that will improve his feeling, his voice and he will breathe more freely. It is not necessary to bleed or purge him until adolescence. If he develops a suppurative lesion, avoid drawing medications.

Directions for the convalescent

Convalescents are men who have enjoyed good health but have become weak. They are like monuments, having suffered insults of weather. They have lost their animation and their blood is impoverished. Take into consideration that if the illness has lasted for a long time, it is necessary to strengthen little by little without hurry; if it has been of short duration, give enough food but in a skillful and progressive manner until improvement is evident. Give them small but very nourishing meals which may benefit them; insist upon their quiet and rest for their limbs are weak; try to lift their spirit through welcome words and pleasant company; give them sweet-scented perfumes and flowers; obtain happiness and music for them; spare them somber thoughts and fatigue. Give them bathtub and Turkish baths of short duration and sitz-baths; massage their limbs with oil. Let there be no violent exercise or strong rubbings so as not to tire them.

Geriatric hygiene

Old people see their strength decline and every day their condition regressing. For them, strong food, in small amounts, in order not to weight down their organs. Purgatives ought not to be used to evacuate bile; leave it in them because it is medicine. It is not necessary to stop the custom of bleeding. After sixty years of age, the plethoric and robust people ought to be bled twice yearly and only in the two seasons (III-58) ; avoid bleeding the cephalic vein and be cautious. When man reaches seventy years of age, change to once a year, no more, and do not use the median vein itself in plethoric people. If he is five years older, it will be only once in two years—two bleedings from the basilic vein. After that age, avoid all bleeding; that may be fatal for the old person. Do not repel surface illnesses to the inside; do not seek too hard to draw them to the surface. Clean their body with perspiration and massages; use fat diets at intervals. Depurate them with emollient foods and keep from imposing drugs upon them.

Management to follow for the one who is ill in only one organ and only at one time

He who is sick at a specific moment ought to be treated before any alteration. Give him a drug opposite to his condition; if the illness persists, continue the same treatment. Treat the one who suffers from the weakness of one organ according to what I have stated about each illness until its cure.

Management to follow for the one who presents with a prodromal symptom

If you discover a prodromal symptom, treat it without waiting for the illness. I have already indicated these premonitory signs. Treat the patient according to the kind of illness and suppress the causes of it.

Chapter II

To Return Health to Patients with Drugs and Dietary Regimens

Now, after having dealt with the preservation of health, I shall speak of the cure of the illness and that is summarized in a single principle: fight the illness with its opposite. The illness due to warmth is treated with cold; it is just the opposite if it comes from coldness. If it comes from moisture, it is treated with dryness and vice versa. Repletion is treated with evacuation at the level of the organs and brain. It is proper to open that which is obstructed and to suppress that which is in surplus (III-59). It is proper to close that which has been opened until it is placed again in good condition (III-60). It is proper to make smooth that which has become rough and vice versa (III-61).

On the different kinds of medications

I shall now mention drugs which expel the humors through stools, those which dominate one temperament, those which make the humor come out, those which alleviate obstructions or which soften, those which burn, those which decompose, those which mature, those which toughen, the astringent, the drawing, the fluidifying, the agitating, those which cause the flesh to bud (III-62), those which scarify. I shall also state their secondary effects and even their tertiary ones.

On purgatives and first about those which evacuate yellow bile

Scammony (III-63) strongly discharges yellow bile; the dose is a third of a drachm; it has a great action on the humors; health is improved by mixing quince (III-64) in it to avoid its harmfulness to the stomach and liver; aloes is administered in the dose of a dinar (III-65) and, then, if necessary, doubling it with drugs such as bdellium (III-66) and gum tragacanth (III-67); yellow myrobalan (III-68) is taken in the dose of an ounce and, likewise, violet (III-69) and also cassia pith (III-70), tamarind (III-71), but not to excess.

That which expels phlegm

One ought to take two daniqs (III-72) of the pulp of colocynth improved with bdellium. Likewise, the donkey cucumber (III-73) which it is also necessary to alter weight for weight with suitable drugs; one also gives some soda (III-74) mixed with salt, a half a drachm of each; that expels all the phlegm; and also two drachms of turpeth (III-75) or twice the amount with food; one can also give at least a drachm of agaric (III-76) and, likewise, seeds of pharbitis (III-77).

That which expels yellow water (III-78)

Use two daniqs of daphnee (III-79) and one daniq of fresh spurge (III-80), one daniq of euphorbia pityusa (III-81) prepared like aloes, a drachm of centaurea (III-82) —all these drugs expel that water.

That which makes black bile come out

Give senna (III-83), fennel (III-84), dodder (III-85), rind of black myrobalan, fumitory (III-86) and a certain amount of borage (III-87) to expel that black bile. A half ounce of all of these drugs obtains this effect. A half drachm of lapis lazuli (III-88) is specific for it; likewise, Armenian stone (III-89) is very energetic in this case.

Constitution and composition of drugs— their primary properties

One ought to administer simple medications as far as judging their effectiveness and to resort to compounds only for the following reasons: when the illness is itself compounded (III-90), it is necessary, then, to alter the medication, giving a sweet food (III-91) and to add it to something to increase its effectiveness if it cannot penetrate; one ought to facilitate its swallowing and, likewise, aid its intestinal transit. If you use a compounded medication, be guided by its composition. Take a mouthful of each purgative drug, count the doses, ignore nothing. Grind with each simple medication whatever may improve it and mix them together; then, divide it into doses. Do the same for all compounded medications; administer it several times in beverages; keep the remainder for later.

On the properties of medications

Medications have primary and secondary active properties and also tertiary properties likely to cause accidents.

The primary properties are warm, cold, dry and moist. I shall begin with cooling drugs.

That which cools, for astringent usage

Of this kind are myrtle (III-92), sumac (III-93), myrobalan, scoria of iron (III-94), emblic (III-95), acacia nilotica (III-96), coral (III-97), balsam (III-98), Armenian earth (III-99), bramble (III-100), arrillus (III-101), bloodwort, gall-nut (III-102), sukk (III-103), choke weed (III-104) mixed with musk (III-105), pomegranate flowers (III-106) mixed with ashes of burned ivory, betel nut (III-107), dry coriander (III-108), cinnamon (III-109) mixed with plantain (III-110): these medications are astringent when used. Galle (III-111), acid beet (III-112), rhubarb (III-113) and barberry (III-114) are cold and astringent.

On simple drugs which warm and do not purge

Be aware that drugs which warm and have not been tried are: soapwort (III-115), incense (III-116), pepper (III-117), cardomom (III-118), capsicum (III-119), saffron, mint (III-120), schoenanthus (III-121), mahaleb (III-122, caper (III-123), artemisia (III-124), nettle (III-125), stavesacre (III-126), organum (III-127), usnea (III-128), styrax (III-129), amber, sweet-scented wood (III-130), the wood called wajj (III-131, melilot (III-132) with dodder, ginger (III-133), gentian (III-134), badaward (III-135), peony (III-136), lacca (III-137), rhubarb, ladanum (III-138), laurel (III-139), germander (III-140), ammi (III-141), sedge (III-142), anethum (III-143), ricin (III-144), glume (III-145), faecula (III-146), madderwort (III-147), myrrh (III-148), marrubium (III-149), sagapenum (III-150), anise (III-151), caraway (III-152) with cumin (III-153), rue (III-154), parsley (III-

155), valeriana (III-156), adiantum (III-157), thyme (III-158), aspalanthus (III-159), galingale (III-160), celadine (III-161), asarum (III-162), pitch (III-163), hyssop (III-164), tar (III-165), feverfew (III-166), balsam, sweet marjoram (III-167) with nettle, corn poppy (III-168), star thistle (III-169), fennel, sweet flag (III-170), chamomile (III-171), nigella (III-172), asafoetida (III-173), pistachio (III-174), sulfur, gum ammoniac (III-175), mustard (III-176), bitumen (III-177), garlic, cubebe (III-178) and costus.

How to recognize moist from dry and the degree of the property of simple medications (III-179)

Every cool or warm medication may be dry or moist. Dryness is recognized by its astringency and moist by what it softens. Physicians differ in opinion as regards the degrees of the property of drugs; I shall enlighten you. The action of the drug which, through reasoning, ought to modify the temperament of the patient represents the first degree of the property. Everything which causes a change hardly perceptible to the senses is a manifestation of the second degree. That which produces a considerable change, without, nevertheless, causing the destruction of the sick organ and does not disturb the temperament, is of the third degree. After this, through its burning heat or by the numbness produced, comes the destruction of the organ; you may say without making a mistake that it is the property of the fourth degree.

On the secondary properties of simple medications which cause maturation

Be aware that every medication which causes maturation is warm and viscous. Its warmth ought to be equal to that of the organ of which you desire the maturation. For example, tallow, pitch, pine resin, oil mixed with wax, oil beaten with warm water, wheat cooked with oil.

On emollient medications

Every medication called emollient is warmer than the organ to be treated but little enough to avoid the dissolution of its tissue. Among these drugs are galbanum (III-180), bdellium, gum ammoniac, styrax and tibial bone marrow from the antilope (III-181).

On medications which harden

They are cold and moist; example: black nightshade (III-182) or water moss (III-183).

On occlusive medications

Everything which is known as an occlusive medication is neither warming nor cooling, does not decompose when in contact with the sick organ and is of the consistency of earth or viscous.

On medications which open

Every medication recognized as deobstruent is incisive and solvent; its taste is like borax (III-184) or bitter, like squill (III-185), bitter almonds (III-186), lily roots (III-187), narcissus (III-188), soda, caper and lupine (III-189).

On cleansing medications

Everything which carries this name is less subtle than the preceding ones; for example, the broad bean (III-190) and among which there are sweet ones like honey and sweet almonds (III-191).

On medications which dilate

Everything you find which widens has a temperate warmth, such as oil of ricin, chamomile, rue and fennel.

On medications which open the orifices of the vessels

Everything known to open the orifices of the conduits as the surgeon would do it has a strong warmth, such as garlic, onion and bile.

On astringent medications

Everything which is useful to close a vessel is astringent without being caustic.

On medications which burn

Every vesicatory medication ought to have an extreme warmth and an extreme density, such as anacard (III-192) and pepper grass (III-193).

On medications which decompose

Every decaying medication possesses a very great warmth and is of a subtle nature (III-194).

On corrosive medications

Medications which gnaw on the flesh are less powerful than the preceding ones, but they scarify and dry wounds.

Drawing medications

Everything which draws is an analogue of the badizahr (III-195) and the purgative. Every medication of this kind is warm and naturally subtle, such as ammoniac (III-196), bdellium or is decomposing because of its warmth like

manure. Antidotes draw be it through their own temperament or through their properties; certain ones act by purg-
ing, others by directly counterattacking. It is not necessary to use them in good health; in this way, the illiterate
make mistakes.

On tranquilizing medications

Medications which suppress pain are warming and
draining towards the outside, cutting and emollient.
Among these medications there are those which numb like
opium and its analogues.

On the tertiary properties of simple drugs

What I shall say of the tertiary properties of drugs, like
the disaggregation of renal concretions, applies to every
solvent and incisive medication which makes things fine or
softens. It never contains any manifest warmth. For example, asparagus roots, cane roots, ground glass and
mahalab; analogue medications possessing a certain
warmth and moisture facilitate expectoration. Those
which have a temperate warmth give juice. That which
provokes expectoration facilitates menstruation. All these
medications are diuretic. The most burning to the taste
are the best.

Method of using medications

After having described the properties and the temperaments of drugs, now, I shall speak of their use. The methods of administration are the oral route and external ap-
plication, such as chartae, pills, syrups, powders, liniments,
ointments, aromatic baths, tattoos (III-197), tinctures,
products of diatomaceous earth, collyria, preserves, bandages, toothpicks, dentifrices, lotions, plasters, powders for
external usage, kohols (III-198), nasal instillation, medi-

cinal drops, that which is used as pessaries, laxatives, washes and fumigants.

Signs and treatments of changes of temperament

Everything which I have reported about illnesses from the scalp to the toe nails may involve the whole body or only one organ. For that which is not accompanied by humoral changes, do not look for their expulsion (III-199). Be cautious! The treatment is to change the temperament of the patient to its opposite. It will be necessary to recognize with wisdom the illness due to the retention of a humor, searching to become familiar with the slightest sign. If the drug causes injury, that means that the temperament of the patient is the same as the medication's. It will be useful, then, to administer the drug opposite to that which caused the illness. The best information is obtained from palpation, the exhaustion of organs, abnormal manifestations of each one of them and excreta. If urine has no sediments, if the pulse is steady, if there is no retention of humors, the illness is not due to them. If pain appears in one place, it means an attack. It is also necessary to consider the age, temperament, color, season, and its characteristics, residence, town, what I have stated about dietetics —all that will aid healing.

Illnesses coming from changes in cold temperament

If the patient has a cold temperament, whatever cools will be unfavorable to him. Everything which warms will be useful to him; his coolness is perceptible by touch, his urine is partially white, his pulse slow to palpation; he suffers neither from thirst nor restlessness and, if that happens to him, it occurs without agitation. If his color is whitish, his flesh flabby, he is old, it is winter in a southern country. If he has already been treated for manifestations of coolness, the evidence is clear. To treat him, use warming medication. Treat hemiplegia similarly.

Illnesses coming from changes in warm temperament

If it is a question of a warm temperament and you treat it with warming medication, that will be harmful. Warmth is recognized by palpation; the urine is red, the pulse regularly rapid. The patient is thirsty, agitated, does not sleep, is thin and his color is yellow. Moreover, if he lives in a southern country, is yellow and it is summer, it is necessary to consider these things. Treat his fever and all his ailments with cold. Let his diet be in harmony with his strength and his appetite.

Symptoms of a bad temperament moist or dry

If the illness comes from one of these temperaments, there are two cases to face: if it is the dry, the patient will present dried; if it is the moist, his flesh will be flabby. The moist will be dried up through cautious management. Whether he be warm or cold at the same time, the dry will be re-established by its opposite. Generally, it is proper to suppress by having to undertake an effective treatment.

Discourse on the illness of plethora and on conditions to observe for evacuation

In case of an illness of plethora, the only remedy is evacuation. Every evacuation ought to be sustained on ten conditions; if they are not united, no evacuation is in order. The first is the examination of the symptoms and let it be only a question of an illness of plethora; then, age, from youth to old age, the custom of bleeding and the strength of the patient; the season, spring or autumn; the general balance of the climate of the inhabited country; the time of day; the warmth or moisture of the temperament of the patient and his florid appearance.

On the kinds of evacuation

Draw from the organ itself what you desire to evacuate from it or from opposing organs or from corresponding ones. Sometimes you will drain the organ in harmony with the illness. Thus, it is that you will place a scarified cupping-glass upon the abdomen to stop a uterine hemorrhage. I have already given the signs of plethora and the medications which drain it.

On illness of the blood in which phlebotomy is indicated and first on the tumor called falgamunia (III-200)

Galen drew blood from a vein in case of the abundance of chyme, when he saw the blood and in case of swelling. In this case, carry out bleeding but only in the sanguineous person; do as he did and bleed as he, himself, bled when you relieve a certain sign of the sanguineous illness. Do it for internal and external illness of the head and joints, for the swelling of the lower part of the ears, in ophthalmia, in the inflammation of the tongue, gingiva, throat and uvula, that of the neighboring zone, the tonsils, in quinsy and colds, pleurisy, illnesses of the lung, those of the kidneys, crural regions, liver, stomach, intestine, anus, spleen, testicles, bladder and kidneys, and also in that of the uterus, umbilicus, in erysipelas and other erythemata.

On bleeding for ulcers and pustules wherever they may be

Do it similarly for ulcers of the head, eyes, pustules, wounds of the ears, for ulcers which run from place to place. Do it for certain illnesses of the intestine and budding tumors. Likewise and in a general manner, bleed for all pustules, wet scab (III-201) from its appearance, for example, in the mouth, on the eyelids and on the flanks.

On the indications for bleeding in vascular plethora and hemorrhage

Bleed in the case of repletion of the vessels, epistaxis and nasal varices, hemorrhage of the teeth (III-202), ears, hemorrhoids, hypermenorrhea and also to evacuate pus, and in varices of the mouth and uterus.

Indications for bleeding for other illnesses

Do it for migraine, vertigo, bad breath, hydrophobia, alopecia; likewise, in the cases of limb contusions, spermatorrhea, joint pains and colds. And also for epilepsy, pannus corneum (III-203), subconjunctival ecchymosis, mature papilloma and lack of appetite, for perineal fistula, sciatica and gastralgia and also for sharp pain and obstruction of the liver.

Treatment of illness of the blood

For these illnesses use the same treatment as for the sunuhus (III-204) : purge of yellow bile after bleeding and for food, rely on the cold ones (III-205). Avoid that which is warming and which increases the amount of blood (III-206). Seek the astringent one, sour (III-207) and acid (III-208) foods. For the knowledge of these illnesses, look for the sign of predominance of the blood. You must cool or dry. That is the act of a skillful and experienced physician.

On illnesses due to yellow bile

Among the illnesses generated by yellow bile are found lientery, mental confusion, hysteria, intermittent fever, sciatica, intestinal hemorrhage, cough, migraine, fluxions (III-209) moving throughout the body, violent pains in the ears, itching of the eyelids, ulcers, joint swellings with pains of some consequence, cracking of the fingers, paronychia, lenticular eruptions, yellow shade of the teeth, crystalgia, syncope, hemorrhage, fistula, jaundice, pustules, small black spots on the skin, obstructions of the liver, abscess of the uterus, pleurisy, dysentery, lack of appetite, vertigo, cracking of the lips, pains of the uvula, cholera, expanding ulcer, dubaïla (III-210), indurated abscess of the anus, pruritus, rubeola, fourmi (III-211), erysipelas and pulmonary ulcer.

On the treatment of illnesses of biliary origin

To treat these illnesses, use what has been previously mentioned for intermittent fever. Expel that yellow bile without bleeding; use cooling agents as for the aforementioned sanguineous illnesses for these illnesses particularly are to be made moist. They are like illness of the blood because of the predominance of warmth; the pains of the patient are the same; gradually look for the signs which allow their separation from the discourse on the predominance of the bile.

On illnesses caused by phlegm

Every patient of this kind has softness as a characteristic. They have hemiplegia, loosening of the flesh, hepatic

migraine, epilepsy, crusted scab, tenesmus, neck tumors
called scrofula, impetigos, loss of memory, painful cold in
the ears, vitiligo, freckles, apoplexy, colds, paralytic twist-
ing of the mouth, elephantiasis, lack of appetite, lice, indurated abscess of the anus, cataract, pupillary dilatation,
offensiveness of the axillae, abdominal illnesses, rectal in-
continence, worms, difficulties in delivery, placental retention, lumbago, diurnal fever, coolness of the spleen or
liver, umbilical hernia and the painful rejection of sanies
(III-212) , joint pains, blackness of the skin, its greenish or
dull shade, dropsy of the uterus, its fleshy tumor, its flatus.

Treatment of illnesses caused by phlegm

It is necessary in these cases to conduct yourself as you
would for moist and cold temperaments, and for that, to
use the signs of predominance of phlegm in the management of the treatment. As for evacuation in these cases, use
drugs given for evacuating bile and after that evacuation,
warm the body; use whatever dries; give a suitable warm
diet. In brief, these illnesses are to be treated by internal
and external warming agents. As for paralysis, it is relieved
with pills of asafoetida and other laxative drugs.

On illnesses caused by black bile

Among the illnesses generated by black bile are warts,
quartan fever, hemorrhoids, epilepsy, cancerous tumor of
the nose, polyps, spasms, abdominal pains, cancer, nevi,
freckles, migraine, restlessness, firm tumors, leprosy, everything which comes from the decomposition of food in the
body, dry cough, flatulency, indurations of the spleen,
melancholia, mental illness, retention of urine, colic,
alopecia, rabies, impetigo, coagulation of milk in the
stomach, the cool liver, rabid hunger, fissures of the anus,

renal and vesical calculi, suprapubic painful swelling, of the abdomen and below the ribs, of the head, ears, ectropion of the eyelids and gout in the foot.

Treatment of illnesses due to atrabile

It is necessary to begin by treating this kind of illness as for leprosy in that it is with drugs. To recognize them, use the signs of predominance of atrabile; evacuate it with the aid of epithyme (III-213) or polypod cuscute. Use warming and moisturizing drugs and your goal will be reached.

Surgical Practice

This comprises three divisions

Now, that I have finished the useful management of treatment, I undertake the manual part. There is, at first, what is done to large and small vessels; then, what is done for the flesh; finally, what is done for bones.

Chapter I

That Which Is Done to Vessels and the Usefulness of Bleeding

Among the vessels, there are those which are bled, others which are ligated and cut. The median vein ought to be opened for every illness of the head and lung, for example, their inflammations. The cephalic ought to be bled with caution in the case of a violent migraine and epistaxis. The basilic for illnesses of the chest or lung. The one which is called median ought to be bled for illnesses of the liver and spleen. In the absence of the basilic, it is necessary to open an arm vein. Open the temple veins in case of permanent head pain; the one which is behind the ears for migraine and ulcers of the head of old people; those which are at the angles of the eyes in case of an occular disease; the one on top of the cranium for head ulcer or tumor; the one of the neck which is specific for leprosy; the one of the forehead in case of an illness of the eye, permanent migraine or tinea capitis; the one of the occiput in case of permanent migraine and dizziness; the one of the tip of the nose in case of maxillary wounds; the sublingual for tumor and ganglions of the neck; those of the knee for any subumbilical visceral illness; the saphenous of the leg for illnesses of the thigh; the sciatic vein in case of sciatic pain; the pedal one for afflictions of the foot.

Technique for incision of arteries

The pulsatile vessels are to be incised in case of migraine and of eye pain when its intensity makes one fear cataract. If a tumor (III-214) is formed after the opening of an artery and the blood does not flow away from it, incise and cut or draw and open it if you wish or extirpate the whole thing. Stop the loss of blood with ligature or cauterization. Afterwards, treat it as a wound until its healing.

Chapter II

Second Division of Surgery

Techniques for the flesh

The techniques for the soft parts are scarification, excision, cauterization, incision. It is scarifications which bleed, others in which it is necessary to aspirate the blood with the aid of a cupping-glass. The blood flows away from the skin in those who have ulcers and wounds. Sometimes non-scarified cupping-glasses are placed with the objective of displacing a humor. Sometimes the cupping-glass is empty; sometimes it contains a tuft of cotton which is set afire to draw the pneuma (III-215) from an organ and also to warm it.

That which ought to be excised

For example, furuncles, warts, and tumors. For the extremities, everything which is susceptible to becoming gangrenous ought to be excised; for example, protuberances of the nose, supplementary digits, webbing between digits, coalesence of the eyelids, the iris if it looks like a grape (III-216), phimosis, pimples of an ulcer which become malignant, a contusion having become gangrenous. Abnormal growths of the tongue and ears ought to be excised as well as the flesh at the level of a piece of glass, an arrow, a fistula, in order to extirpate them all; and also the breasts of the male (III-217), varices of the legs, hemorrhoids, fistulae, the blackish greasy elements of a wound, gangrenous flesh, that which lengthens the uvula, everything sprouting on the gingivae, the vessel of Medina (III-218) and everything closing the ears or growing on the white of the eye, the pterygium, mulberry (III-219), ectropion, subungual granuloma, the penis of the hermaphrodite and umbilical hernia, the black parts of the prepuce and everything closing the anus; even excise everything which seems useful to you to suppress and similarly everything coming to the outside; suture the wound or let a scar form.

On cauterization

You will have to cauterize every part of the body to stop an arterial hemorrhage there or following a wound of the large vessels of which the drainage of blood disturbs the physician. One ought to cauterize to dry moist organs and to drain flabby flesh, to warm the cold body and to arrest old drainage areas.

On incision

One incises to cause the bad humor to leave, the pus of an abscess, decomposed blood of a hematoma, cataract, hailstone (III-220), water in the head (III-221), nodules, the calculus which must be extracted, every moveable gland, morphea (III-222), every bubo. One incises for dropsy, hydrocoele, fleshy hernia.

Chapter III

On Bone and Principally on the Repair of Fractures

All you may do to the bones is to repair their fracture or reset them. To repair a fracture, it is necessary at first to carry out reduction, prepare the fragments to retake their place, to cut down the wounding points—that is the correct method. Afterwards, place a suitable bandage, not too tight, not too loose; little bandages ought to begin being placed in the middle, then, one can tighten down to the correct position. Finally and especially, prepare wrapped and well-arranged splints. Give the wounded person a light diet at first, then a heavy diet so that he may become strengthened. From the beginning fear warm inflammation for the wounded person because the blood carries it there. With all your might prevent the arrival of blood at the site of the wound with the aid of any cold therapeutic agent which will repel it. Forbid any movement until complete healing. Insist upon the wounded one's patience to sustain this immobilization.

Treatments of dislocations

The dislocation is treated by traction until the dislocated bone retakes its place after which it will be necessary to restrain it for a certain period of time. You will order astringent drugs and an acid diet until certain that inflammation will be avoided as well as the formation of a hematoma. The least amount of time for healing is a month, sometimes ten days longer.

Behold the entire account of practical medicine! Here I conclude my purpose—I have finished.

4

Extant Bibliography of The Poem

(11, 26, 27, 34, 46, 52)

1. Incipit translato Canticorum . . . cum commento
   Averoys facta ab Arabico in Latinum a Armangando
   Blasii. 341 fol. Venetiis, per P. Maufer et Soc., 1483.
2. *Ibid.,* 1484.
3. Avicennae Liber Canonis de Medicinis Cordialibus
   et Cantica cum castigationibus Andreae Alpagi Bel-
   lonensis . . . Fol. Venetiis apud Juntas, 1544.
4. Avicennae Cantica ex arabico in lat. translata, Venetiis, 1552.
5. Avicennae Liber Canonis de Medicinis Cordialibus et
   Cantica olina Gerardo Carmonensi, Venetiis, 1555.
6. Avicennae medicorum Arabum principis, Liber Canonis de Medicinis Cordialibus et Cantica. Jam olim
   quidem a Gerardo Carmonensi ex arabico sermone in
   latinum conversa. Nunc autem demum a Benedicto
   Rinio Veneto, philosopho er medico eminentissimo;
   hic acceserunt, Avicennae libellus de removendis nocumentis quae accedunt in regimine sanitatis, ejusdem
   tractatus de syrupo acetoso, ab eodam Alpago ex
   arabico in latinum sermonen translati. Basileae. Per
   Joannes Heruagios, 1556.
7. Avicenna, Libri in re medica omnes, lat. redd. a
   Gerardo Cremonensi et A. Alpago, ex. recogn. A. J. P.
   Mongii et J. Costaei et cum eorundem annotationibus
   id est libri Canonis V, de viribus cordis, de removendis
   nocumentis in regimine sanitatis, de syrupo acetoso et
   Cantica, 2 voll. Venetiis Valgrisius, 1564.

8. Avicennae Opera omnia; Venetiis, apud Juntas 1595 in 2 voll. I. Tabulae Isagogicae in Universam medicinem, collectae et editae A. Fabricio Rapsano d. Chirugico. II. Arabum Medicorum principis Ex. Gerardi Cremonensis Versione et Andreae Alpagi Bellunensis Castigatione.

9. Avicennae Arabum medicorum principis, ex Gerardo Cremonensis versione et Andreae Alpagi Bellunensis castigatione. A Joanne Costaeo et Joanne Paulo Mongio annotationibus iampridem illustratus, Venetiis 1608.

10. Canticum principis abi-alis, Ibn Sinae, vulgo dicti Avicennae, de medicina, seu breve, perspicuum et concinne digestum institutionum medicorum compendium cui adjecti aphorismi medici Jo. Mesnaei Damasceni, ex arabico latine reddita ab Ant. Deusingio . . . accessit hujusce Oratio de felicitate sepientium. Groningae, ex. off. Jo. Nicolai, 1649.

11. Undated: Avicennae Canonis libri V ex Gerardi Cremonensis versione et Andreae Alpagi Bellunensis, castigatione, a Joanne Costaeo et Joanne Paulo Mongio annotationibus jampridem illustratus, nunc cero ab eodem Costaeo recognitus . . . Libellus Viribus cordis, translatus ab Arnoldo de Villanova. Libelli de Removendi Nocumentis et de Syrupo acetoso, traducti ex arabico in latinum per Andream de Alpago, Bellunensem, Cantica translata ab Armengando Blasii. Vita ipsius Avicennae ex Sorsano arabe, ejus discipulo, a Nicolae Massa latine scripta . . . Additis nuper etiam librorum Canonis oeconomiae nec non tabulis isagogicis in universam medicinam es arte Humain id est Joannitti Arabis, per Fabium Paulinum, Utinsem . . . collectis a Fabritio Raspano . . . cum indicibus quatuor.

12. Arabic and Latin manuscripts may be found in the following libraries:
   a) Algiers (1752).
   b) Beirut (289).
   c) Berlin (6268).
   d) Bibliothèque du P. Sabath (782).
   e) Bodléiene, cat. Uri (527_2, 645, 1254) ; cat. Nicool (333_1).
   f) British Museum (8933; 801 incomplete).
   g) Calcutta, ed. 1829.
   h) Escorial, cat. Derembourg (788_{12}, 853_2).
   i) Leipsiz (463).
   j) Leyde (1325).
   k) Lucknow, ed. 1845.
   l) Lugd (721, 722, 723, 726).
   m) Madrid (336).
   n) Paris (3038_3, 2943_2).
   o) Vindob (292).

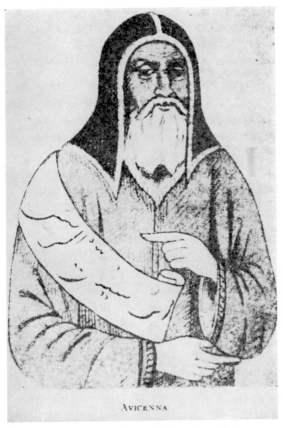

AVICENNA

Avicenna: the Chief, the Teacher. (Taken from Reference no. 31.)

5

Conclusion

*A*VICENNA'S main purpose in compiling this work was to create a practical guide which students had to learn by rote and which the Master would develop in the course of his lessons (26). In his endeavor to make medical truth available in its purity to other physicians (44), the philosopher-physician attempted to expound upon the fundamentals of the art of medicine in a simultaneously clear and succinct manner (40).

It is obvious that Avicenna's scientific medicine is based upon the theories of the *pneuma* and the elements evidenced throughout ancient medicine as well as upon the humoral doctrine of Hippocrates and the theory of therapeutics of Galen (12, 24, 26, 30). To these, he appended observation and the experimental method which he employed to some extent. Further, Avicenna had no doubts about his theories, demanding absolute authority in all medical matters and claiming that its totality should constitute an immutable law (12).

As a philosopher of science, the Prince of Physicians strove to understand the whole of positive knowledge (44). He acquired an extensive acquaintance with the science of his time (33) and through his profound intellectual capabilities he developed a philosophy and precepts of medicine which are very similar to our modern concepts of the Art (48). In addition, he became an astute clinician whose search for the principle laws of medicine caused him to impose upon himself and his followers a systematic and comprehensive method which is too often disregarded in today's over-specialized and anti-intellectual world (38). As the *Poem* demonstrates, his advice to other physicians on approaching individuals and their illnesses probably brought him more than satisfactory *rapport* with his patients. Avicenna relied upon his powers of observation as seen in his description of pulses and upon the study of materials excreted from the body to obtain a complete clinical picture of any patient. Among his more remarkable contributions to medicine are his recognition of the Guinea worm (53) and of the dangers of smoking, his interpretation of the specific gravity and sediments of urine, his awareness of benign and malignant diseases as well as of functional ailments and his innovation that obstetrics and pediatrics are important entities which deserve special consideration within the realm of general practice. Nevertheless, it may be observed that the physician-philosopher did not completely ignore the ideas of antiquity that astronomical bodies influence the course of disease and the destiny of human life.

It has been helpful to obtain an idea of the drugs mentioned in the *Poem* from the works of Flückinger, Hanbury and Rezzaq (21, 42). Avicenna listed one-sixth of the drugs which he described in *al-Qānūn* (6), many of which it has been found impossible to identify (51). Although he continued insisting upon the treatment of disease according to Galen's theory of opposites, the Prince of Physicians believed in using only pure drugs. Furthermore, he reserved compounding of medications solely for very specific reasons, an idea held by many physicians today.

The *Poem of Medicine* remains among Avicenna's major works which demonstrate his avid desire for thoroughness and a fervent dedication to truth (22, 38). Because of these attributes in addition to his indisputable universality, the Prince of Physicians will continue to occupy his rightful position among those few remarkable individuals recorded in the history of the Middle Ages.

Notes

I

1. This map represents a composite of the approximate itinerary followed by Avicenna from bibliographical entries nos, 1, 11, 15 and 19.
2. In A. D. 622, Muhammad and his followers emigrated from Mecca to Medina and this "hegira" (Arabic *hijra*, flight) became the starting point of the Muslim era (6, 11, 30).
3. Avicenna's full name, in literal translation, means: Father of 'Alī, the Horse, the Son of the Servant, of the Prophet, the Son of Sina (39). His own name was really al-Ḥusain, a name shared with one of the two grandsons of Muhammad; his name of "honor" was Abu 'Ali (Father of 'Alī), shared with the Prophet's cousin and son-in-law, the fourth caliph of Islam. 'Abd-Allāh was the name of Avicenna's father, a name identical to that of the Prophet's father. Sīnā was the name of his great-grand-great-grandfather (25, 49).
4. *Al-Qānūn* may also be translated as "the Law" (22, 33). This is probably nearer to the correct meaning Avicenna intended to imply with this great work. *Al-Qanūn* was finished in the city of Iṣfahān (20).
5. It has been a difficult task to find out how Avicenna acquired the title of Prince of Physicians. It is evident that such a title was awarded by his contemporaries because of Avicenna's erudition (5). However, one encounters the translation of *al-Sheikh al-Ra'is* as: the Chief Master (7, 43), the Chief of Chiefs (18, 39), the Sheik, the Chief (30), the Chief of Lords (17), the Prince of Scholars (35), the Prince (of science), the Teacher (*par excellence*) (22). The literal translation of the two words is

"the Chief, the Teacher." It is probable that our concept of this man as the Prince of Physicians comes from the Latin scholars' having referred to him as *arabicum medicorum principes*. This title was most certainly not given to him by H. G. Wells as was purported by bibliographical entry no. 33. Still another title has been granted to Avicenna by his national supporters, that of *al-Muallimu' l-Thani* (the Second Teacher). Who was the first? Certain authors have claimed Muhammad (39), Hippocrates or Galen (18) to be the first. However, more authorities agree that the "First Teacher" was probably Aristotle (17, 29, 43, 50).

6. One author claims that this lady may have been Avicenna's wife (1). On the other hand, two authorities of two different centuries disagree, one stating that this lady was a means to an end in that Avicenna received his position through her (52) and the other one claiming that by the age of twenty-five, Avicenna had already married a girl of his native town and had two sons (54).

7. This brief account of Avicenna's life was compiled from the following bibliographical references: 1, 4, 6, 7, 8, 9, 10, 11, 13, 14, 16, 20, 22, 25, 28, 29, 30, 31, 32, 38, 39, 44, 45, 46, 48, 49, 52, 53 and 54.

The dates encompassing the life of this physician—philosopher are not as exact as one would like them to be. It may be concluded that he was born sometime between 979 and 985 (11, 54) in the month of Ṣafar which corresponded to our August and that he died between the ages of 56 and 58 (1, 38, 46) in the month of Ramadhān which corresponded to a period bridging June and July of 1037 A. D.

The cause of his death was probably due to that indicated in the text of this book. Yet, another author claims that Avicenna developed a colonic carcinoma (16).

8. *Inferno*: IV, 142:   Euclide geomètra e Tolomeo
                         Ippocrate, Avicenna e Galïeno

Averroès, che 'l gran comento feo (2).
(Euclid the geometer and Ptolemy
Hippocrates, Avicenna and Galen
Averroes who made the great com-
ment.)

II

1. The lines of this composition are similar to what we know as iambic pentameter (36, 47). Each verse consists of two such lines separated by a hemistitch.

III

1. Elements: earth, fire, air and water.
2. Kingdoms: animal, vegetable and mineral.
3. That which would constitute an illness which results from imbalance or from a conflict between two of them.
4. Of all the elements.
5. Zendj: tribes of Moors of Southern Morocco.
6. Temperate zone.
7. Muscle.
8. Imagination.
9. Semolina: the finest wheat flour.
10. Oxymel: a mixture of honey and dilute acetic acid used as an excipient.
11. Garlic: a wild tuberous plant which is used for tumors, antiseptic, drainage of menstrua and the after-birth, cold and phlegmatic temperaments, paralysis, chronic cough and lung afflictions, decreasing the sexual appetite, and topically for snake and rabid dog bites.
12. Henbane: a fetid herbal, *Hyoscyamus niger,* which has medicinal properties similar to belladonna.
13. Muscles: ?Bell's palsy.
14. Of an organ with a lumen.
15. Sometimes perceived and sometimes imperceptible to palpation.
16. Done with four fingers.

17. Rapid and constant, rapid and intermittent, slow and constant, slow and intermittent.
18. Temperate zone.
19. Saffron: from Persia and Asia Minor, this substance possesses a sugar, essential oils and croncin, a red powder; it is used to treat juvenile aphthae, lentigo, vitiligo and impetigo; it strengthens the stomach, liver, heart and viscera, beautifies the skin and is used as a diuretic and aphrodisiac.
20. Cassia fistula: dried pods of the drumstick tree of India used as an emollient, gargle for pharyngitides, for relaxing the uterus and in jaundice.
21. Murri: an acid flavored condiment prepared with wheat, barley and mashed fish; it acts as a detergent, clearing the chest, lungs and gastrointestinal tract of bad humors; it aids sciatica.
22. Bloodwort: a deep-red coloring matter in roots of resinous quality; it has a sweetish, pungent and burning taste and contains benzoic acid; it mainly fortifies the stomach, arrests hemorrhage and diarrhea; it is noxious to the kidneys without tragacanth.
23. A gas.
24. Between white and yellow.
25. Probably desquamation of the ducts.
26. Dysentery.
27. Of humors.
28. Of vessels or organs.
29. Migraine, intense thirst, restlessness.
30. Epidemic.
31. That of the house of death.
32. Mars and Saturn.
33. Sun and Jupiter.
34. *al Qānūn* (the Law) = rules: *v.* note 1-4.
35. Lientery: a diarrhea in which food is discharged imperfectly digested.
36. Temperate.

37. Simoon: dry, hot, violent wind laden with dust.
38. Francolin: partridge specifically from Southern Asia.
39. Zirabaj: meat soaked in vinegar.
40. An unknown substance.
41. Leek omelettes: made from an onion-like bulb, *Allium porrum*.
42. Hulame: a veal dish.
43. Qaris: a lamb dish.
44. Tifsil: lentil soup.
45. Masus: meat preserved with sour wine.
46. Costus oil: a volatile oil obtained from the fragrant root of the annual herb *Sausaurea lappa* which is a native of Kashmir; it is used as a preservative and in perfumes.
47. Pea size.
48. Purslane juice: juice from the leaves of portulaca plants which resemble moss rose.
49. Fenugrec: an extract of the seed of this plant is given for abdominal colic and head wounds and with honey as an aphrodisiac.
50. Yellow amber: this substance is useful for stopping bleeding, palpitations, lung and stomach humors, nausea, diarrhea and tenesmus.
51. Aloes: a lilaceous plant of Africa which has a pleasant odor and minute proportions of a violatile oil; its bitter resin is used as a purgative and may be compounded with other drugs; it is a native of the Caspian region and Samarcand.
52. After-birth: placenta, umbilical cord and aminiotic sac.
53. Savin: a fruit which is used for gangrene and hemorrhoids.
54. Sulfur: of four kinds, red, yellow, gray, and black, sulfurs are employed for gale (?eczema) and as abortives.
55. Colocynth: sometimes called bitter-apple, this powerful cathartic is distributed widely throughout Ceylon, Persia, Arabia, Syria and Egypt; it is sometimes compounded with aloes and scammony.

56. This line #916 of the Arabic manuscript of Jahier and Noureddine should really precede #931, which has been done in this interpretation.

57. Poppy: probably refers to the immature fruits of *Papaver somniferum* var. *album* of Persia of which the milky juice contains opium.

58. Spring and autumn.

59. Worms in the abdomen, an extra finger, cataract.

60. Diarrhea with astringents.

61. Trachea made rough with coughing; stomach made smooth through disease.

62. Vesicating.

63. Scammony: a root resin which has no taste but which leaves an acrid sensation in the throat following its ingestion; it is found in Asia Minor, Syria and Southern Russia; it is a markedly active cathartic especially when used with colocynth.

64. Quince: this substance strengthens and increases the tone of the stomach, stops diarrhea, vomiting, hemoptysis and menstrual flow and is a diuretic.

65. Dinar: the exact size and weight of this coin are unknown.

66. Bdellium: a blue and black gum resin like myrrh of a plant of the genus *Commiphora;* it is used to treat snake bites, renal and vesical calculi and to increase the flow of urine, sperm and milk.

67. Gum tragacanth: a gummy exudate from the *Astragulus* found in Asia Minor and Persia; it is a useful additive for medicines in which its action is that of a demulcent.

68. Myrobalan: several kinds of dried astringent fruits, somewhat like a prune, from which tannin is obtained; it aids the stomach, teeth and gingivae and is helpful in jaundice, hemorrhoids, palpitations, splenic and digestive infections.

69. Violet: an extract is used to resolve atrabiliary illnesses, intestinal inflammations and cephalalgia.

70. Cassia pith: this substance resembles cinnamon bark and has an essential oil of which the odor is suggestive of Ceylon cinnamon; it is found in Asia and India; the most probable use is that of an alimentary tract stimulant.
71. Tamarind: of Indian origin this type of date preserved in sugar is used as a mild, cooling laxative or fever drink; it has an agreeable and refreshing taste.
72. Daniqs: the exact size and weight of these coins are unknown.
73. Cucumber: this is employed to reduce fevers and for diuresis.
74. Soda: the white salt, $Na_2CO_3 \cdot 10\ H_2O$, used as a salt replacement; it drives away bitterness and colors the skin black if taken excessively; it is used for tremblings, convulsions and paralysis.
75. Turpeth: a purgative root with a whitish cortex of a tropical Asiatic vine, *Convolvulus turpethum.*
76. Agaric: a toadstool-mushroom-like plant, *Agaricus oreades,* which emits hydrocyanic acid; it is used in hepatic disturbances, asthma, cough, dysuria, renal disorders and jaundice.
77. Pharbitis: the seeds of this plant have cathartic action and possess a nutty taste which subsequently becomes disagreeable, leaving a presistent acridity; it is found in India.
78. ? ascites.
79. Daphnee: a resinoid substance from the bark of the spurge laurel located in Siberia; as a liniment it has both purgative and vesicatory effects; it is employed as a sudorific and is useful in veneral, rheumatic and scrofulous complaints.
80. Spurge: *v.* euphorbia pityusa.
81. Euphorbia pityusa: a member of cactus-like plants from Morocco which produces an acid, amorphous resin which is used medicinally as an emetic and purgative.
82. Centaurea: this substance is useful for dropsy and icterus.

83. Senna: of Arabian origin, these yellowish-green leaves have a tea-like odor but are without marked taste; they are used in a nauseating infusion as a purgative.
84. Fennel: a perennial Indian herb of which the aromatic seeds contain a bitter-sweet essential oil; it is used as an aphrodisiac, diuretic, emmenagogue and a desobstruent for the liver, kidneys and bladder; it is used in fevers, against rabies and as a lactogenic agent.
85. Dodder: a rootless and leafless parasitic plant used to resolve hepatic and renal obstructions, to protect the vessels and pelvis from bad humors and to strengthen the stomach and liver.
86. Fumitory: of the genus *Fumaria,* this plant is known for its antiscorbutic action.
87. Borage: a rough, hairy, black flowered herb which is used as a demulcent and diaphoretic; it fortifies the heart, combats inflammation of the oral cavity and reduces anxiety.
88. Lapis lazuli: an azure-blue powder, presumably containing iron pyrites; it is probably the sapphire of the ancients used for curing melancholia, asthma and warts.
89. Armenian stone: earthy blue cupric carbonate which is used in melancholia, convulsions, epilepsy and insanity.
90. Due to two humors, etc.
91. Honey.
92. Myrtle: from Malay and Java, the leaves of this tree have cajuptol which is a bluish-green oil with a camphoraceous odor and a bitter aromatic taste; it is used as an internal stimulant, antispasmodic and diaphoretic and as an external rubefacient.
93. Sumac: a tree with red, acid berries in Turkey of which a decoction of leaves is employed in chronic diarrhea, abdominal pains, prophylaxis of ocular variola and suppurative otorrhea.
94. Scoria of iron: these are crude minerals containing iron which are used to dry the humors, dissolve warm tumors and fortify the stomach.

95. Emblic: an East Indian tree like myrobalan which closes and fortifies the stomach.

96. Acacia nilotica: a gum from the thorny tree of the Nile valley which is used as an adjuvant rather than a medication.

97. Coral: a species of marine vegetables which expands the chest, aiding respiration, and strengthens the heart.

98. Balsam: an aromatic fluid or oleoresin of the Gurjun tree of India; it contains gurjunic acid which is like the hydrate of abietinic acid and which stimulates mucous membranes especially those of the genitourinary organs.

99. Armenian earth: a soft, clayey, bright-red soil which stops hemoptysis, hemorrhage, bubonic plague, aids wounds, catarrhal dyspnea, asthma, phthisis and counteracts the pain of hemorrhoids.

100. Bramble: the fruit of this plant is useful against intestinal ulcers, diarrhea, hemoptysis, erysipelas, wounds, renal and vesical calculi and hemorrhoids.

101. Arrillus: this is used to stop diarrhea, hemoptysis, palpitations and nausea.

102. Gall-nut: from Asia Minor and Syria, it is a parasitic swelling containing insect eggs which were placed in the bark of a tree punctured by the adult insect; it contains gallotannin and tannic acid, a free sugar, resin and protein; it is used externally as an astringent and internally for chronic cough, uterine contractions, intestinal ulcerations and oral pathology.

103. Sukk: a substance purported to purify and fortify the viscera and to cure infantile diarrhea.

104. Choke weed: a root of a parasitic herb with obscure uses and effects.

105. Musk: a viscid, chocolate colored fluid which is obtained from the abdominal sac of the male musk deer; when powdered, it has a powerful odor and bitter taste, fortifies limbs, adds palpitations of the heart and a cold temperament and is a carminative, tranquilizer and an antidote for poisons.

106. Pomegranate flowers: known for their astringent properties, they correct oral bleeding, hemoptysis, ulcers and diarrhea.
107. Betel nut: a product of a tropical Asian palm of which the active principle remains ill-defined; when powdered, it is used specifically to eradicate tapeworms.
108. Coriander: this substance is used to cure inflammatory tumors, scrofula and to decrease sexual potency.
109. Cinnamon: a native of Ceylon, this substance is employed as a stimulant and carminative, fortifying the stomach and combating edema and jaundice; its active principle is mainly cinnamaldehyde.
110. Plantain: widespread throughout Egypt, Arabia and India, this plant produces light pink to gray seeds which are without taste or odor but which contain considerable quantities of mucilage; it is used as a cooling demulcent drink in cases of chronic diarrhea, a scarring agent for burns and tumors and in asthma, cough, hemoptysis, edema, hemorrhage of hemorrhoids and for quartan and tertian fevers.
111. Galle: this substance is used to calm chronic cough, intestinal ulcers and to strengthen weakened and softened organs.
112. Acid beet: a type of wild beet with sour juice which is purported to cure ulcers and be helpful in thirst, jaundice, nausea and febrile palpitations.
113. Rhubarb: from Tibet and Asia, the root of this plant contains calcium oxalate besides being bitter, astringent and nauseous; it is used as a purgative, stomachic and tonic.
114. Barberry: this substance is derived from dried barberry roots of the genus *Mahonia* which contain the bitter alkaloids of berberine, oxyacanthine and berbamine; it is used as a tonic, febrifuge and antiperiodic.
115. Soapwort: from the Old World pink family *Caryophyllaceae* which contains the starch compound saponin, it is used in plasters.

116. Incense: this is employed in stomach disorders, palpitations and diarrhea.
117. Pepper: this familiar substance is useful against viscous phlegm, colic, abdominal distention, chronic cough, skin diseases and in hastening conception.
118. Cardamom: a seed from India and Ceylon which contains a turpentine-camphor and fatty and essential oils; it is pleasantly aromatic and is used to fortify and warm the stomach and liver, as an antinauseant and as a secretory agent.
119. Capsicum: the pungent and fiery seeds of chillies or peppers of Indian and African origin which are used as a rubefacient, local gargle and gastro-intestinal stimulant.
120. Mint: a plant from Asia which emits a fragrant odor when rubbed and has a pungent aromatic taste because of its essential oil content; it is used as a stimulant, diuretic and emmenagogue and for throat pain, snake bites, orthopnea, colic and sciatica.
121. Schoenanth: of Indian origin, this substance is the oil of ginger grass known as citronella oil obtained from the flowers of the plant; it is used medicinally in rheumatism, for the growth of hair and internally as a carminative for colic; an infusion of the leaves possesses diaphoretic properties.
122. Mahaleb: a type of cherry from Arabia which is a small red inedible fruit used for renal and vesical calculi, drainage of urine, colic and iliac pains and as an antinauseant.
123. Caper: a prickly shrub of the Mediterranean area, this plant has flower buds and berries which are pickled and used in sauces; a tea is also made from the plant; it is used as an emetic and for indurations, scrofula, hepatic and splenic disorders.
124. Artemisia: this is a thistle herb of which the flowerheads contain one percent of an essential oil called wormseed (cymene-camphor) and which grow on the steppes of the Kirghiz and Northern Turkestan; the unopened flower-

heads are used as an anthelmintic especially in *Ascaris* infestations.

125. Nettle: a coarse herb of which the seeds are used against renal and vesical calculi and as an aphrodisiac.

126. Stavesacre: from Asia Minor these seeds have a bitter taste and produce a tingling sensation to mucous membranes when chewed; the fatty oil obtained from the seeds destroys body pediculi; its content of delphine, an alkaloid, makes the plant highly poisonous; it is used internally in neuralgic conditions and externally against impetigo and pox.

127. Origanum: aromatic mints probably related to wild, sweet marjoram.

128. Usnea: a Persian bush-tree moss.

129. Styrax: a soft, viscid resin-like honey, grayish-brown in color which has a disagreeable odor and a burning aromatic taste, being sharply pungent; its chief constituent is cinnamylic cinnamate; its use is that of expectorant and stimulant in chronic bronchial infections; it is present throughout Asia Minor.

130. Sweet-scented wood: probably aloes (*v.* III-51).

131. Wajj: a substance for stomach, liver, splenic and colic ailments, ruptures, uterine tumors, tongue ailments, vitiligo, leprosy and nervous conditions; it is also an aphrodisiac and diuretic.

132. Melilot: sweet clover seeds of the genus *Melilotus* which are helpful in convulsions, epilepsy, testicular disorders, edema, uterine infections, headache and inactive stomachs.

133. Ginger: from a native plant of Asia, the volatile oil has an agreeable aromatic odor and the resin has a burning taste; it is used as a stomachic and with other medicaments.

134. Gentian: bitter roots which are used as a tonic and stomachic; it is of Southern European origin and is useful in hepatic and splenic ailments, vitiligo, aids menstruation and is a diuretic.

135. Badaward: obtained from a very heavy black wood, this

substance is employed as a diuretic and in renal and splenic afflictions.

136. Peony: this acrid white flower is used to combat viscous phlegm and cough and to warm nerves and tendons.

137. Lacca: a resinous substance secreted by a scale insect *Tachardia lacca* which lives on the twigs of various trees; it is used in hypochrondia, palpitations, icterus, dropsy and for splenic, renal and vesical afflictions.

138. Ladanum: a soft, dark oleoresin with a fragrant odor and bitter taste from the rockrose species *Cistus ladanum;* it is used as a dilating agent for cough, asthma, ear infections and inflammatory tumors.

139. Laurel: the chopped leaves of this tree from Asia Minor and Persia contain bitter almond oil; they are used in making cherry laurel water which has an aromatic odor and a bitter taste; it is used for hepatic and splenic tumors, facial tics and paralysis and for animal bites.

140. Germander: a member of the genus of herbs *Lamiaceae* used against intestinal worms.

141. Ammi: a small genus of annual herbs from India and Egypt which has minute spicy fruits; the aromatic volatile oils consist of thymol and cymol and have a burning taste; it is used as a carminative for colic, a diuretic and for chest suppuration, leprosy and impetigo.

142. Sedge: edible tuberous roots with obscure medicinal actions.

143. Anethum: an Asiatic herb, *Anethum graveolens,* which has aromatic foliage with a lemon-like odor; it is used as a carminative and stomachic.

144. Ricin: a white amorphous, violently poisonous protein of the castor oil bean with an acrid, bland taste from Algeria and Egypt.

145. Glume: a scaley leaf grass of unknown medicinal properties.

146. Faecula: a starch.

147. Madderwort: a red tropical plant of the *Rubiaceae*

which opens hepatic and splenic obstructions, acts as a diuretic and is used as emmenagogue, abortive and suppository.

148. Myrrh: an aromatic gum resin with a bitter, acrid, pungent taste with a peculiarly agreeable fragrance from Egypt and Arabia; it is used as a stimulating tonic but has no real medicinal powers.

149. Marrubium: old world mints resembling horehound; it is a diuretic and emmenagogue, opens hepatic and splenic obstructions and purifies the lung.

150. Sagapenum: a pinkish-brown resin from Persia with an alliaceous odor and a bitter taste; like galbanum, it contains umbelliferone, 7-hydroxy-coumarin; it is used as an expectorant and for the preparation of plasters.

151. Anise: from Egypt, this essential oil has a sweetish aromatic taste; it is used as a carminative, stimulant and as an adjunct to other medicaments.

152. Caraway: the seeds contain nine percent of a volatile oil, carvene and carvol; the plant grown in Persia, Armenia and Morocco is employed as an aromatic stimulant.

153. Cummin: a dwarf plant of the Nile, Arabia and India which produces aromatic seeds with a strong aromatic taste and odor of caraway; it is used in curry powder, but its medicinal value is questioned.

154. Rue: a strong-scented perennial woody herb, *Ruta graveolens*, of which the bark is used for dyspepsia, dysentery and chronic diarrhea.

155. Parsley: a mountain plant which is used against dropsy.

156. Valeriana: the root of the garden heliotrope with a camphor-like odor and a bitter aromatic taste; it is used as a stimulant, antispasmodic, diuretic, emmenagogue and antipleuritic.

157. Adiantum: the maidenhair fern of the family *Polypodiaceae*; it combats calculi, viscous humors of the lung (asthma), jaundice and dysuria.

158. Thyme: this pungent aromatic seasoning prossesses an

essential oil which is deep reddish-brown in color; the active constituents are thymol, cymene and thymene; as a medication it is used as a local disinfectant, liniment and external stimulant; the Iberian Peninsula is its origin.

159. Aspalanthus: a thorny, South African shrub of the pea family *Fabaceae* which possesses a fragrant oil; its wood acts on pustules, purulent ulcers and all organs and cures headaches and hemorrhoids.

160. Galingale: a pungent aromatic rhizome oil from India related to ginger; its active principle is galangin, a yellowish material; it is used medicinally as a dentifrice and pain reliever and fortifies the reproductive organs.

161. Celandine: a biennial herb, *Chelidonum majus,* of the poppy family *Papaveraceae* which is supposed to cure warts, jaundice and eye diseases.

162. Asarum: a rhizome of the acaulescent herbs which has a pungent, bitter taste and an aromatic odor; it is employed in hepatic and splenic obstructions, jaundice, edema, sciatica and chronic rheumatism.

163. Pitch: this dry substance is used to dry up harmful humors, to soften indurated and scrofulous tumors and to rid fingernails of white spots.

164. Hyssop: aromatic, pungent mint leaves which are used for bruises; they purify the lungs, act against chronic cough and asthma, evacuate phlegm and intestinal gas.

165. Wood tar: made from Asian trees, this substance serves as an ointment for cutaneous diseases; as a water infusion, it is taken internally.

166. Feverfew: made from the roots of chrysanthemums, this medication from Asia possesses febrifugal qualities; it has a slight aromatic smell with a persistent pungent taste which leaves a tingling sensation of the mucous membranes; it is a sialogogue and is used for the relief of toothache and as a stimulant and rubefacient.

167. Sweet marjoram: a fragrant herb used in dysuria, colic,

melancholia, edema, facial tic, headache and ear obstructions.

168. Corn poppy: this plant, *Papaver rhoeas,* possesses papaverine and one percent opium; medicinally, it is a smooth muscle relaxant, an analgesic and a local anesthetic.

169. Star-thistle: sometimes called knapweed, *Centaurea calcitrapa,* it reduces fevers and is a dessicant.

170. Sweet flag: the pungent rootstock of *Acorus calamus;* it is used for colic, ruptures, uterine tumors, vitiligo, leprosy and as an aphrodisiac and diuretic.

171. Chamomile: a blue essential oil made from the flowerheads of a Persian plant; its apple-scented, bitter medicinal principle has antispasmodic and diaphoretic properties; it is also used as a bitter stomachic, tonic diuretic and emmenagogue.

172. Nigella: black seeds of perennial herbs of fennel flowers, *Nigella sativa;* it is used as an anthelmintic.

173. Asafoetida: a perennial umbelliferous plant of which the darkly colored gum resin has a strong alliaceous odor which is somewhat repulsive and has the taste of garlic; it is used primarily as a stimulant and antispasmodic.

174. Pistacho nut: from Bukhārā, this nut is good for nausea, colic, snake bites and hepatic and pulmonary infections.

175. Gum ammoniac: a Persian gum resin from the ammoniac plant which possesses a bitter-sweet, nauseating acrid taste; it is used as an expectorant, stimulant and in certain plaster preparations.

176. Mustard: this familiar substance is employed to attract phlegm.

177. Bitumen: a tar-like substance from the Sea of Sodome or the Black Sea with an offensive odor used externally.

178. Cubebe: a dried, unripe, nearly full-grown fruit of *Piper cubeba* of which the oleoresin is used to treat gonorrhea; it is smoked for nasal catarrh.

179. Each medication had certain degrees (°) of the four basic temperaments.

180. Galbanum: this substance is similar to asafoetida and is native to Northen Persia; it is a brown gum resin with a volatile oil, possessing an aromatic odor and unpleasant taste; it is used as a plaster for swellings and as a stimulant and expectorant.

181. Bone marrow: this is useful as a carminative, a softening agent for indurations and muscle, tendon and ligament deformities and for vaginal disorders.

182. Black nightshade: from Asia minor, this plant possesses a poisonous foliage and edible blackberries; also known as petty morel, its medicinal value is related to the action of belladonna-like alkaloids.

183. Water moss: a member of the genus *Fontinalis* of aquatic algae, mosses and liverworts, *F. antipyretica* possesses a quality suggested by its name.

184. Borax: a native of Tibet, $Na_2B_4O_7 \cdot 10\ H_2O$ is used as an antiseptic and flux.

185. Squill: a bulbous herb with a mucilaginous, bitter, acrid taste from India and Asia Minor; it is used as a diuretic and expectorant and contains physiologically active glycosides which cause it to be a cardiac stimulant.

186. Bitter almonds: these are used for lung infections, dry cough, renal afflictions, hepatic, splenic and ear obstructions and as an aphrodisiac.

187. Lily root: this substance from Africa is like aloes and is used as a purgative.

188. Narcissus: an Old World bulbous herb which is used for the treatment of epilepsy, burns and pustules and as an emetic.

189. Lupine: from the region of the Caspian Sea and Siberia, the seed of this plant was used for food in early times; an essential oil extracted from the seeds has the odor of hops and a bitter, acrid taste; it is used as an anthelmintic and as an astringent.

190. Broad bean: this substance swells in the alimentary tract and is difficultly digested; it is used for slowing the pulse, suppressing the appetite and as an aphrodisiac.

191. Almonds: these nuts come from Egypt and Palastine and contain a sweet essential oil identified as benzaldehyde; they are used for lung diseases, dry cough, to purify the kidneys and bladder, to relieve hepatic and splenic obstructions and as an aphrodisiac.
192. Anacard: a fruit of the plant of the sumac family which aids intelligence and the activity of the human mind.
193. Pepper grass: also known as golden cress, *Lepidium sativum* has pods with a pungent flavor; it is used for gastric and splenic discomfort, in dysuria and as an aphrodisiac.
194. An example would be arsenic.
195. Badizahr: origin of the world "bezoar;" it is purported to possess antidotal properties.
196. Ammoniac: a gum resin with resorcin from Africa and Lybia which resembles myrobalan and emblic in action.
197. Tattoos: to disguise an element of the skin.
198. Kohols: highly rectified spirits.
199. Functional disturbance.
200. Falgamunia: phlegmon.
201. Oozing eczema.
202. Teeth: probably gingivae.
203. Pannus corneum: a vascular tissue causing a superficial opacity of the cornea occurring especially in trachoma.
204. Sunuhus: a continuous fever due to bubbling of the blood.
205. Lettuces, pears, tamarinds.
206. Meats, sweet things, pungent spices.
207. Sour grapes or gooseberries.
208. Vinegar and tamarinds.
209. Fluxions: excessive flow of blood toward any organ.
210. Dubaïla; a painful abscess full of thick decomposed material within the body.
211. Fourmi: a small pustule with swelling which becomes an ulcer.
212. Sanies: a thin, blood-tinged, seropurulent fluid discharged from ulcers or infected wounds.

213. Epithyme: this substance is somewhat like thyme; it evacuates atrabile.
214. Probably an aneurysm.
215. Pneuma: breath or vital spirit.
216. If it herniates.
217. Probably in case of gynecomastia.
218. The tumor due to *Dracunculus medinensis.*
219. Papilloma.
220. Probably chalazion.
221. ? hydrocephaly.
222. Morphea: small black vascular tumors of the skin, ? allied to scleroderma.

Bibliography

1. Afnan, S. M.: *Avicenna: His Life and Works.* London, George Allen & Unwin Ltd., 1958. Pp. 295.
2. Alighieri, D.: *La Divina Commedia.* Firenze, G. Barbèra, 1902. Pp. 623.
3. Alverny, M. T. d'.: Les traductions d'Avicenna. *Accad. Lincei. Q. 40:*71–90, 1957.
4. Ardalan, A. G.: What Avicenna means to the Persians. *Bull. New York Acad. Med., 31:*302–306, April 1955.
5. Baas, J. H.: *Grundriss der Geschichte der Medizin und des Heilenden Standes.* Stuttgart, V. von Ferdinand Enke, 1876. Pp. 904.
6. Bishop, W. J.: Avicenna, prince of physicians. *Pharm. J., 118:*357–358, May 1, 1954.
7. Browne, E. G.: *Arabian Medicine.* Cambridge, University Press 1921. Pp. 139.
8. Browne, E. G.: *A Literary History of Persia.* Vol II. London, Cambridge University Press, 1928, Pp. 521.
9. Boucetta, O.: Ibn Sina (Avicenna): sa vie, son oeuvre médicale. *Maroc méd., 36:*185–190, 1957.
10. Campbell, D.: *Arabian Medicine and Its Influences on the Middle Ages.* Vol. I. London, Kegan Paul, Trench, Trubner and Co., Ltd., 1921. Pp. 208.
11. Carra de Vaux, B.: *Avicenna.* Paris, Felix Alcan, 1900. Pp. 302.
12. Castiglioni, A.: *Storia della Medicina.* Vol. I. Verona, Arnoldo Mondadori, 1936. Pp. 509.
13. Chatard, J. A.: Avicenna and arabian medicine. *Bull. Johns Hopkins Hosp., 19:*157–160, June 1908.
14. Cohen, H. M.: Avicenna—Avenzoar. (980-1200 A. D.). Fifth of a series of essays on the history of medicine from

the earliest times. *Maryland M. J.*, *52*:321–327, August 1909.

15. Czerminski, A.: *Avicenna*. Warszawa. Wiedza Powszechna, 1953. Pp. 102.

16. Dawson, J. B.: Avicenna, the prince of physicians. *M. J. Australia, 2*:751–755, December 15, 1928.

17. Elgood, C.: *A Medical History of Persia and the Eastern Caliphate from the Earliest Times Until the Year A. D. 1932*. Cambridge, Cambridge University Press, 1951. Pp. 617.

18. Elgood, C.: *Medicine in Persia*. Clio Medica XIV. New York, Paul B. Hoeber, 1934. Pp. 105.

19. The epic of medicine VI: Arabian medicine. *M D Medical Newsmagazine, 4*:99–123, April 1960.

20. Finot, A.: Le millenaire d'Avicenne. *Presse méd., 62*:845, May 29, 1954.

21. Flückinger, F. A., and Hanbury, D.: *Pharmacographia: A History of the Principle Drugs of Vegetable Origin Met With in Great Britain and British India*. London, Macmillan and Co., 1874. Pp. 682.

22. Gabrieli, G.: Biografie et bibliografie di scienziati arabi: Avicenna. *Arch. stor. sc., 4*:258–270, 1923.

23. Galdston, I.: Avicenna and islamic science. *Bull. New York Acad. Med., 31*:300–301, April 1955.

24. Grunner, O. C.: The interpretation of Avicenna. *Ann. Med. Hist., 3*:354–358, Winter 1921.

25. Gürkan, K. I.: *Ebu Ali Ibn-i Sina*. Istanbul, Sermet Matbiasi, 1954. Pp. 80.

26. Jahier, H., and Noureddine, A.: *Avicenne: Poème de la médecine; Al-Husayn Ibn 'Abd Allah Ibn Sina: 'Urguza fi'ṭ-ṭibb; Cantica Avicennae. Texte arabe, traduction française, traduction latine du XIII*ᵉ *siècle avec introduction, notes et index*. Paris, Société d'Edition "Les Belles Lettres," 1956. Pp. 209.

27. Jahier, H., and Noureddine, A.: Cantica avicennae version latine de l'*Urguza fi'ṭ-ṭibb* d'Avicenne. *Cah. Tunis, 3*:41–48, 1955.

28. Klein, S.: *De Avicenna Medico*. Vratislaviae, Typis Leopoldi Freund, 1845. Pp. 27.

29. Leclerc, L.: *Historie de la Médecine Arabe*. Vol. I. Paris, Libraire des Sociétés Asiatiques de Paris, etc., 1876. Pp. 587.

30. Levy, R.: Avicenna—his life and times. *Med. Hist., 1*:249–261, July, 1957.

31. Lichtwardt, H. A.: Avicenna—philosopher and genious, teacher and surgeon. *J. Michigan M. Soc., 49*:568–572, May 1950.

32. Major, R. H.: *A History of Medicine*. Vol. I. Springfield Illinois, Thomas, 1954. Pp. 563.

33. Mostafavi, J.: Avicenna: the "prince of physicians" introduced. *Acta med. iran., 1*:104–123, Fall 1956.

34. Naficy, S.: *Bibliographie des Principaux Travaux Européens sur Avicenna*. Teheran, Imprimerie de l'Université, 1953. Pp. 30.

35. Nizamuddin, M.: A sketch of Avicenna as a scientist. *Indian J. Hist. Med., 2*:21–26, 1957.

36. Opitz, K.: Avicenna: das Lehrgedicht über die Heilkunde. *Quellen Gesch. Naturwiss. Med., 7*:304–374, October 1939.

37. Osler, W.: *The Evolution of Modern Medicine*. New Haven, Yale University Press, 1921. Pp. 243.

38. Pope, A. U.: Avicenna and his cultural background. *Bull. New York Acad. Med., 31*:318–333, April 1955.

39. Price H. W.: Some notes on Avicenna. *Hist. Bull., 7*:5–8, November 1942.

40. Renaud, H. P. J.: Trois études d'histoire de la médecine arabe en occident. III.—Une suite à l'*Urguza* d'Avicenne sur la médecine: Le poème d'Ibn 'Azrun et ses commentateurs. *Hesperis Rabat, 12*:204–228, 1931.

41. Rey, P.: La pensée médicale et philosophique d'Avicenne. *Praxis, 48*:472–476, May 7, 1959.

42. Rezzaq ar-Djezairy, d'Abd ar-: *Kachef ar-rounmoûz*. Translated by L. Leclerc. Paris, J. B. Baillière et Fils, 1874. Pp. 398.

43. Sa'di, L. M.: Glimpses into the history of arabic medicine. *Bull Med. Libr. Assoc., 46*:206–218, April 1958.
44. Sarton, G.: Avicenna—physician, scientist and philosopher. *Bull New York Acad. Med., 31*:307–317, April 1955.
45. Shah, M. H.: Avicenna—his life and works. *Hamdard Med. Dig., 2*:1–6, July 1958.
46. Soubiran, A.: *Avicenne, Prince des Médecins, sa Vie et sa Doctrine.* Paris, Librarie Lipchutz, 1935. Pp. 176.
47. Temkin, O.: *Avicenna: Poème de la médecine. Bull. Hist. Med., 31*:380–381, July-August 1957.
48. Ünver, A. S.: Aphorisms of Avicenna. *J. Hist. Med., 14*:197–201, April 1959.
49. Wickens, G. M., ed.: *Avicenna: Scientist and Philosopher.* London, Suzac and Co., Ltd., 1952. Pp. 128.
50. Wilczynski, J.: Contribution oubliée d'Ibn-Sina à la théorie des êtres vivants. *Arch. Int. Hist. Sci., 7*:35–45, 1954.
51. Wootton, A. C.: *Chronicles of Pharmacy.* Vol I. London, Macmillan and Co., 1910. Pp. 428.
52. Wüstenfeld, F.: *Geschichte des Arabischen Aerzte und Naturforscher.* Göttingen, Vandenhoeck und Ruprecht, 1840. Pp. 167.
53. Zaki-Ali.: Neuvième centenaire d'Avicenne, prince des médecins. *Bull. Soc. Fr. Hist. Méd., 32*:215–221, 1938.
54. Zeki, M.: *Avicenna and His Age.* Baghdad, The Times Press, 1952. Pp. 22.

Index